Communic with Patient

Brent D. Ruben,
Rutgers Univer

KENDALL/HUNT PUBLISHING COMPANY
2460 Kerper Boulevard P.O. Box 539 Dubuque, Iowa 52004-0539

27073392

5-97

S0-CRO-534

This edition printed directly from camera-ready copy.

Copyright © 1992 by Brent D. Ruben

ISBN 0-8403-7430-5

Printed in the United States of America
10   9   8   7   6   5   4   3   2   1

When you meet your friend on the roadside or in the market place, let the spirit in you move your lips and direct your tongue.

Let the voice within your voice speak to the ear of his ear;

For his soul will keep the truth of your heart as the taste of the wine is remembered.

When the colour is forgotten and the vessel is no more.

Kahlil Gibran, *The Prophet*

Table of Contents

Preface

In my work with physicians and paramedical professionals, three frequently asked questions are:

> "Is communication really all that important? I am a physician (or a nurse, dentist, pharmacist, or X-ray technician). I went to school to be a clinician, not a public relations specialist!"

> "Is communication really all that difficult? I'm an educated individual, and I lead a successful life personally and professionally. I have been doing so for a number of years. Could I really have done all this if I didn't know how to communicate effectively?"

> "Isn't what it takes to be successful in communication just common sense? Is it really necessary to spend time thinking about communication theories and concepts?"

These are reasonable and important questions, and essentially this book is dedicated to addressing them. At this point, I will but briefly comment on each question as a prelude to the more detailed discussions in the pages ahead.

<u>Communication is vital in health care.</u> Communication understanding and competence is an important component of many, if not most, occupations. In none is it more important than health, where quality care depends upon both clinical/technical competence on the one hand and communication competence on the other.

<u>Successful communication is a difficult activity.</u> One need only consider the problem of achieving international understanding, the high divorce rate, or the challenge we each face in our own organizations and personal relationships to realize that communication can be an extremely difficult process. Health communication is among the most challenging types of communication because of the many barriers that must be overcome.

One does not automatically acquire an understanding of the communication process or the interpersonal skill naturally necessary to these challenges. Moreover, these abilities do not necessarily emerge as a result of higher education or professional experience.

<u>Communication understanding and competence requires *uncommon* sense.</u> While some of what it takes to be successful may be thought of as common sense, this alone does not take us very far when it comes to communication. Common sense, for instance, may tell us that other people are very much like we are, and that their perspectives, concerns, and information needs are similar to our own. This may be the case in some instances, but in the case of communication between caregivers and patients, *<u>uncommon</u>* sense – which leads one to question what would otherwise be taken for granted – is by far the more appropriate strategy.

Communicating with Patients is written with these questions and the issues they raise, in mind. Specifically, it is intended to meet three goals: 1) To provide a summary of current perspectives on the role of communication in caregiver-patient encounters and relationships; 2) to provide a overview of relevant health communication theories and concepts; and 3) to provide a practical framework for analyzing and enhancing encounters with patients.

Acknowledgements

Many people have played a role in the refinement of the ideas presented in this book. First, I want to thank those who contributed to the evolution of *The Bottomline: A Patient Relations Training Program,* which I initially developed in 1985. I would particularly like to acknowledge the assistance of June Bowman, now Vice President of Nursing at Centennial Medical Center in Nashville. Then in the capacity of Director of Training and Management Development at Morristown Memorial Hospital in Morristown, New Jersey, June played an indispensable role in helping to test, refine, and promote *The Bottomline.* For her encouragement and professional guidance, I continue to be deeply grateful. The vision and support of Brian Grissler, Senior Vice President and Chief Operating Officer at Morristown Hospital during the period was also invaluable.

Others whose contributions figured importantly in the early development of *The Bottomline* were Frank Chimielinski of Johnson & Johnson; Linda Lederman, a friend and colleague at Rutgers University; and Bruce Dalstrom, former Vice President for Personnel at Morristown Hospital. Acknowledgement is also due to W. David Burns, Assistant Vice President for Student Life at Rutgers; Robert Bierman, Director of Medical Services at the Rutgers University Health Services; and David Christensen, former Administrator of the Rutgers Health Service.

Much of the inspiration that led to my involvement in the health and medical communication came as a result of my appointment to the National Institutes of Health Advisory Board. Gratitude is expressed to Secretary of Health and Human Services, Richard Schweiker, and my former colleagues on the Digestive Diseases Advisory Board, especially Suzanne Rosenthal, President of the Coalition of Digestive Disease Organizations; Tom Almy, Distinguished Professor of Medicine, Veterans Administration Medical and Regional Office Center, White River Junction, Vermont; Harold Roth, former Director, Division of Digestive Diseases and Nutrition, National Institutes of Health; Thelma Thiel, Executive Director, American Liver Foundation; Paul Sherlock, M.D., former Professor and Chairman of the Department of Medicine, Memorial Sloan-Kettering Cancer Center; Harry Tamoney, M.D.; and Ralph Bain, former Executive Director of the Advisory Board.

I am also grateful to a number of people at Johnson & Johnson Hospital Services for their support of my work in the area of caregiver-patient communication, among them Denis Hamilton, Victoria Strohmeyer, Regis Karch, Phil Doyle, and Peg Bowers.

Special thanks to Rob Robinson and Denise Juliano at Merck Sharp & Dohme for their enthusiasm and encouragement.

Certainly much of what I now understand about the problems and prospects of caregiver-patient communication, I learned from caregivers themselves. I want to express my sincere appreciation to the dedicated physicians, nurses, administrators, patient representatives, pharmacists, therapists, receptionists, transporters, food service personnel, housekeeping staff, and others with whom I have had the pleasure of working over the course of past seven years at Humana Health Care Plans, Overlook Hospital, Humana Hospital-Metropolitan, Goddard Medical Associates, West Virginia University Medical School, Yale University Health Service, Columbia-FreeState Health System, The Rehab Hospital of York, St. James Hospital, Cathedral Healthcare System, Humana Hospital-Sunrise, Rutgers University Health Service, Chilton Memorial Hospital, Morristown Memorial Hospital, St. Clares-Riverside Medical Center, Mountainside Hospital, West Virginia University Health Service, Pittsburgh University Health Service, and Duquesne University Health Service.

Perhaps I should most thank the nearly 4,500 patients whose questionnaire and interview responses have given me – and other professionals, paraprofessionals, and support staff members with whom I have shared these thoughts – a deeper understanding of the patient perspective on the health care experience.

Finally, to Nurit Guttman, Jann Ruben, John Chabrak, Gary Kreps, Donna Timko, Gary Kreps, Walter Zakahi, Todd Hunt, Carol Briggs, Monica Marciczkiewicz, and Robbi Ruben who have provided assistance at various phases in my work on this project, and to Paul Cardi of Kendall-Hunt Publishers, my sincere thanks.

Brent D. Ruben
Belle Mead, New Jersey

Chapter 1

INTRODUCTION

One of the many changes in the health care environment is the increasing emphasis being placed on the patient and his or her satisfaction as a recipient of health care services. The concern with the quality of patient care is certainly not a new one. However, the focus on patients as consumers – who can and do make decisions within the health care marketplace – represents a significant shift with a number of important implications for the 1990s and beyond.

In this opening chapter, the primary objective is to explore some of the basic implications of the growing emphasis on the patient's perspective on health care.

Patients Often Equate Communication Competence with Clinical Competence.

One might hope that patients would assess the quality of their health care using the same standards caregivers apply. If this were the case, a patient's level of satisfaction would closely correspond to a provider's assessment. Caregivers could then focus their attention exclusively on providing the best possible clinical and technical care, and positive patient assessments would naturally follow. However, as we shall discuss in some detail later, evidence suggests that patients generally look at health care experiences in quite a different way than caregivers do. As a result, patients often use different criteria and arrive at different conclusions when they evaluate their experiences (Ruben, 1990a, 1991, 1992b; Ruben & Bowman, 1986).

Most patients and visitors to a hospital, HMO, clinic, private practice, geriatric center, or other health care facility do not have the medical knowledge to validly assess the quality of the medical care provided. They do make assessments, however, and they tend to do so based primarily on the communication and relationship skills of the caregivers with whom they come in contact.

Caregivers' assessments reflect a medical perspective, and are based on the appropriateness of diagnosis, treatment, and the technical and clinical competence provided by a health care

1

team. Patients' assessments, on the other hand, are based largely on <u>communication competence</u> – on the ability of caregivers to convey a sense of professional competence, interest, concern, and caring. Thus, when someone says: "I have an excellent physician or dentist" or "The hospital (or HMO, clinic, geriatric facility, or practice) is excellent" they are, in all likelihood commenting more on the communication competence of the health care providers than on their technical and clinical competence. The implication is that caregivers must be as concerned about their communication and relationship skills as they are about their technical and clinical skills in order to gain the recognition and respect they deserve from their patients. Moreover, as we shall discuss in some detail later, interpersonal competence contributes not only to patient satisfaction, but also to higher quality health care.

Every Staff Member Contributes to Patient Care

From the medical perspective, the phrase the "health care team" refers primarily to physicians, nurses, and other professional health care providers. Yet to many patients – and even more so to family and friends – everyone with whom they have contact is a potentially significant member of the team. Each has the potential to contribute meaningfully to their satisfaction or dissatisfaction with a health care service or facility, and each can have an impact on the the overall quality of the patient's, family member's, or visitor's experience. Therefore, a lack of interpersonal skill or sensitivity by clerical, support, service, security, or maintenance staff can have as significant and lasting an impact as the clinical care provided by physicians or nurses (e.g. Ruben, 1990a, 1990b; Ruben, Guttman & Christensen, 1992).

Everything a Staff Member Says and Does Matters

The quality of patients' experiences and the impressions they form and remember begin with the expression on the face of a receptionist or the tone of voice of the telephone operator. Every contact with staff members provide additional verbal and nonverbal messages which help to define the outlook a patient, family member, or visitor takes with him or her upon departure.

Quality Communication and Relationships Are Vital

For Patients

Caregiver-patient communication is a complex and difficult process. Scientific studies document these difficulties, as do reports of everyday experiences of many patients and caregivers. In one study, researchers found that in 47.5 per cent of the caregiver-patient encounters studied, the session ended with neither the patient nor the caregiver receiving the message the other was most concerned with conveying (Wertz, Sorenson & Heeren, 1988).

Staff interpersonal skill and sensitivity are important to client, customer, or guest satisfaction in nearly all business and organizational contexts. In no other setting, however, is the need for interpersonal communication competence as great as in health care.

For most people health problems are very frightening. Even situations that are "routine" for health care staff are likely to be a "crisis" for a patient and his or her family. Health care facilities themselves can be anxiety-producing places for many. Uneasiness and discomfort resulting from learned associations are often intensified by unfamiliar equipment, confusing terminology, and the presence of persons who are ill or disabled.

In some circumstances, the quality of communication between caregivers and patients – and among members of the health care team – can have life-and-death consequences. All things considered, the significance of interpersonal competence and sensitivity in caregiver-patient encounters cannot be overemphasized.

Interpersonal skills by physicians, nurses, and other staff can contribute positively to health care in a great many respects, including better compliance with the recommended treatment, greater patient satisfaction with medical services, more appropriate use of patient-care services, better adjustment to chronic disease, and in some instances, a favorable impact on the course of disease and rate of recovery. And as indicated earlier, caregiver communication competence is likely to be the primary factor upon which most patients base their overall assessments of the quality of care, the caregiver, and the caregiver institution.

For Caregivers

Most individuals who select careers in health care do so because of a strong desire to help others. No satisfaction is greater than that which derives from the sense that one has made a difference to the life of another. Quality interpersonal communication and relationships – with patients and colleagues – can be as vital to the satisfaction of staff as it is to that of patients.

For Health Care Institutions

In today's environment, the prosperity of any health care institution – and in turn the well-being of its patients and staff – is contingent upon maintaining viability in a dynamic and highly competitive marketplace. Relations with patients – and among staff – is key to this success. As with any product or service business, consumer satisfaction is essential to a positive image within a community, to repeat business, to referrals, and to survival and growth for the organization.

Every encounter with health care personnel provides the basis for messages which collectively create the impressions patients, family members, and visitor form. In this respect, effective patient relations is directly related to the facility's financial "bottom line."

Quality Communication and Relationships
Do Not Occur Naturally

Communication competence is not an inherited capability, nor is it a capacity that necessarily accompanies a higher education or professional training. In fact, it can be argued that as a person becomes more technically educated and specialized, he or she can more easily relate to individuals with similar backgrounds, yet has greater difficulty communicating comfortably and effectively with others who lack this common ground.

In stressful health care positions – especially those involving a high level of repetitive communication – the natural state of affairs is to gradually become numbed to the experiences of patients. The result even for the most dedicated health caregiver is a gradual deterioration in interpersonal sensitivity and in the ability to empathize with the patient's perspective. An appreciation of the nature of caregiver-patient communication and its role in establishing relationships can be useful in reinforcing and regenerating declining interpersonal sensitivity and skill. Moreover, this same awareness and skill can improve communication with coworkers.

Critical Incidents in Caregiver-Patient Communication

The clinical meaning of the term critical is well-known. Circumstances can also be "critical" from a communication perspective. Such events are often not life-threatening but they may jeopardize the quality of health care nonetheless. Consider the following reported cases:

- After weeks of pain and visits to several physicians, a patient has been referred to a highly-regarded neurologist. The patient introduces herself and begins to describe her problem. The neurologist explains that it isn't necessary to hear her symptoms, that the examination and test results will tell him everything he will need to know.

- A pediatrician at an HMO clinic listening to the chest of a two-year old child with flu symptoms turns and casually comments to the parents who he has never seen before, "Did you know your child has a hole in the heart? It's probably a VSD."

- A 38 year-old is considering a vasectomy, has a number of questions and concerns, and schedules a consultation visit with a urologist. When he asks about possible side effects, the physician responds "There's really no evidence to suggest that there are negative side effects, but who knows. We thought Thalidamide was safe, too." The patient says he has some concerns about the procedure. The physician hands him a pamphlet "which will answer all the questions," and tells him to call the receptionist to schedule the procedure if he decides to go ahead.

- A health care administrator speaking to a group of new rehabilitation patients recovering from strokes begins by telling them: "Strokes are the third most common cause of death in the U.S. Each year 500,000 people have strokes; 200,000 of these die. So, you all should consider yourselves lucky!"

• While conducting a Doppler echocardiogram on an adolescent boy, the technician and cardiologist carry on a technical discussion of a patient "with a big heart." The first reference by the technologist is to "the boy with the big heart." As the exchange continues, the two begin to refer to the patient simply as "big heart." The adolescent leaves wondering whether he was "big heart."

• The son of a geriatric patient writes to his mother's physician to confidentially share his concern that his mother's health is deteriorating despite her claims to the contrary. He explains to the physician that in recent months his mother has begun denying and understating her health problems. The son notes that while she will probably tell the physician that she's eating well, in actuality, her average evening meal consists of two alcoholic beverages, a cigarette, and perhaps some hors d'oeuvres. When the mother arrives for her next appointment with the physician, he reads her the letter sent by her son, and asks if all this is true. The mother is devastated.

• A patient and his family is waiting to be seen. They overhear a physician speaking angrily to a technologist and a nurse about an "echo" that was conducted on the wrong patient.

• A patient who had previously been operated on for breast cancer discovers several new lumps and a cough which her oncologist describes to her as "suspicious." Her physician sends her to a nearby X-ray group for chest X-rays, and says he will contact her later that day or early the next to discuss the results. At the radiologist's office the X-rays are completed, and the woman is asked to return to the crowded waiting room while the film is developed. In ten minutes, the receptionist walks into the still-full waiting room, catches the patient's eye, and announces loudly across the room: "The doctor has developed the X-rays, and has spoken to your physician. . . . He wants you to take the X-rays and go <u>immediately</u> to the Emergency room of the hospital. He'll meet you there.

Each of these situations is a critical incident from the perspective of communication and relationship quality. In every case, there is a loss . . . of confidence, trust, information, and of the potential for quality health care. This occurs not for the lack of good intention, nor of first-rate <u>clinical</u> skill, but rather for the lack of <u>interpersonal</u> skill.

These are the kinds of stories that patients and family members tell perhaps dozens of times to neighbors, friends, and colleagues over the course of days, weeks, or even years. Incidents such as these not only compromise health care; they also damage the reputations of caregivers and institutions, and plant the seeds out of which malpractice litigation may later grow. For all of these reasons, it is important to understand what it is that makes communication encounters critical for patients, and what can be done to prevent negative outcomes.

Chapter 2

HEALTH CARE IN THE 1990s –
A SIGNIFICANT CHALLENGE

Images in the Public Media

There is little question that health, health care, and health caregivers are topics of great public interest and concern. Major articles and feature sections on various aspects of health appear regularly in newspapers and magazines across the country, and the topics of health care and the health care system are routinely the focus of television and radio news and talk shows.

Recent headlines of media features on health care include:

"Ten Ways to Choose a Doctor and What to Look for"
USA Today

"Studies Reveal Widespread Abuse of Medical Students During Education"
Chronicle of Higher Education

"New R_x Success Put Into Practice: McDoctor"
Des Moines Register

"Sick and Tired: Uneasy Patients May Be Surprised to Find Their Doctors Are Worried Too"
Time

"Physician's Placing More Emphasis on Ads"
New York Times

"Physicians Should Examine Their Watches"
USA Today

"Pick a hospital you like, like you would buy a car. . . Shop around"
Good Morning America

Even a cursory review of the articles and broadcast segments underscores three points:

1. Health care is receiving increasing attention in the media.

2. The image of health care presented in the media is overwhelmingly negative.

3. The advice provided to readers – directly or indirectly – is leading to more critical, skeptical, questioning, and demanding patients; and this in turn will present a greater challenge for health care administrators, professionals, support, and service staff at all levels in institutions of all types.

Against this backdrop it is not surprising that a Louis Harris Poll determined that eight of nine citizens believe the U. S. health care system needs a major overhaul (*USA Today*, May 25, 1989). Growing discontent regarding health care, health care personnel, and our health care systems in general is widespread, and detractors are becoming increasingly visible and vocal.

Even physicians, traditionally immune to harsh public criticism, have fallen victim to the tide of discontent. According to author Nancy Gibbs (1989) writing for *Time*: "To judge by the popular press . . . too many physicians who are not magicians are charlatans. Though somewhat less extreme, the results of a survey reported in *Good Health Magazine* indicate over roughly half of those surveyed agreed with the following statements regarding physicians:

"Doctors don't care about people as much as they used to."

"Doctors usually don't explain things well to their patients."

"People are beginning to lose faith in their doctors."

Consistent with these findings are results from a Yankelovich Clancy Shulman study which reports that large segments of the public are dissatisfied with physicians' medical care, diagnoses, caring, listening, punctuality, and fees (Gibbs, 1989).

In the present climate physicians, too, are understandably frustrated, and the challenges they face are substantial.

The air of the operating room, where once the doctor was sovereign, is now so dense with the second guesses of insurers, regulators, lawyers, consultants and risk managers that the physician has little room to breathe, much less heal. Small wonder that the doctor-patient relationship, once something of a sacred covenant, has been infected by the climate in which it grows. (Gibbs, 1989)

A Time of Change

Few fields have undergone the rapid and pervasive change that has characterized health care in recent years. The combined impact of social, political, and technological change, and most especially the changing economic developments, has been dramatic. And, in turn, these changes have had a major impact on health care workers at all levels.

A number of factors have contributed to the present situation. Among these are:

- Cost pressures
- More demanding consumers
- Capital and labor shortages
- Increasing competition
- Rapid technological change
- Litigation
- HIV/AIDS and substance abuse
- Concerns regarding quality of health care and health care system
- Breakdown in caregiver-patient relationships

Our focus here will be on the last two of these factors: concerns regarding quality of care and issues related to a breakdown in caregiver-patient relationships.

The Issue of Quality Health Care

The topic of "quality" is widely discussed in a variety of contemporary contexts. A great number of industries have become concerned – even obsessed – with improving the quality of the manufacturing, marketing, distribution, and management processes. What *Business Week* terms "the quality imperative" emphasizes evaluating performance, simplifying tasks, monitoring competition, improving efficiency and, especially, increasing customer satisfaction.

Parallel concerns and concepts are increasingly apparent in health care. As in other fields, quality can't be taken for granted. Moreover, in today's health care environment, caregivers and administrators cannot be content with knowing themselves that quality care is provided at their institution. Patients and their families must also have this confidence.

If a person has a satisfying experience with a particular hospital, HMO, clinic, or physician, there is every reason to suppose that he or she will choose the same health care provider in the future. Conversely, the dissatisfied individual is likely to use other caregivers for subsequent care. The dissatisfied patient is also likely to tell friends, neighbors, and associates about his or her dissatisfaction. Such patients are likely to talk about their experience to many more people than patients who are satisfied with the treatment they receive. The result is that dissatisfaction and negativism multiply rapidly within a patient group or a community. This multiplier effect can have a dramatic impact on the reputation and image of a caregiver or health care institution in a remarkably short period of time.

Clinical and Technical Quality

In analyzing the challenges of quality facing health care providers, primary attention is understandably focused on clinical/technical aspects of care, and we are seeing increasing efforts to gather, quantify, and analyze information on clinical outcomes. One large project of this kind is sponsored by the Joint Commission on Accreditation of health care Organizations (JCAHO) and involves about 400 hospitals (McCormick, 190, p. 34). There are many other substantial initiatives in this area as well. The Humana group, for example, collects and analyzes data from each of its member hospitals relative to claims, readmission rates, infection rates, complication rates, and length of stay for 14 clinical departments. System-wide profiles are then fed back to the individual institution as a baseline for quality assessment (McCormick, 190, p. 35).

Administrative Quality

Emphasis is also being directed toward questions of administrative quality – matters related to management procedure and policy. Attesting to the growing interest in administrative quality is the emergence of programs such as Phillip Crosby Associates' Quality Improvement Process (QIP), and 3M's Total Quality Management (TQM) both of which apply quality assurance methods from other industries to the health care field.

Relationship Quality

As central as clinical/medical and administrative practices are to the quality of health care, much of the discontent with the quality of care has less to do with clinical or administrative quality than it does with what might be termed *relationship* quality. As we will discuss in more detail in Chapter 3. Research by confirms that much of the widespread public dis-satisfaction is the result of a lack of quality in caregiver-patient relationships (e.g. Ruben, 1990a, 1990b, 1992b; Omachonu, 1990; Ben-Sira, 1990).

To the extent that relationship quality is one of three basic components of the health care quality equation, increasing attention can and should be directed toward caregiver-patient interpersonal communication and relationship enhancement. Initiatives with this objective can enhance:

- Patient satisfaction
- Health care quality
- Marketing and public relations efforts
- Organizational development and team-building
- Management and staff development
- Quality assurance and risk management
- Practice building and enhancement

Chapter 3

PATIENT PERSPECTIVES ON THE QUALITY OF CARE

"We tend to overlook patient perceptions in stressful, busy, hectic times. If we put ourselves in their place, it allows us to stand back for a moment and reassess the situation.
                    Emergency Room Nurse, Humana Hospital–Sunrise, Las Vegas, NV

Imagine yourself in the following situation:

You are 55 years of age. You work at staying in pretty good shape; you've never been hospitalized a day in your life. For the past four weeks you have had symptoms of the flu with a headache, sore throat, and cough. The first week you spent a couple of days at home taking aspirin, and you seemed to get better. However, the cough has lingered along with a feeling of shortness of breath. Finally at your wife's insistence you make an appointment for Friday morning.

The physician's exam seems to go well. He listens to your chest and tells you he wants you to have a chest X-ray which he states he will look at himself. Following the X-ray you wait in the waiting room for almost an hour. Finally the nurse calls you and leads you back into the physician's office.

He's sitting behind the desk writing on a pad. He tears off the top sheet and hands it to you saying:

"Here is a prescription for an antibiotic. Get it filled and take it for the next ten days. The X-ray shows a small spot on your left lung - about the size of a 25 cent piece. I'm not sure what it is. I read the X-ray wet. We'll take another X-ray in 10 days and see if there are any changes. In the meantime, I suggest you stay home from work for a few days, get plenty of rest, and take the medication. Any questions? No, well fine I'll see you in 10 days."

As you stumble to the car your anxiety begins to mount. You replay his words: "Spot on the lungs," "The size of a 25 cent piece," "Don't know what it is."

11

You've known people around you who have had cancer, but you never really thought about this being a possibility for you. Maybe you have it. You try to tell yourself not to worry, to have a positive attitude. The spot – if there even is one – could be something other than cancer. But in the back of your mind you're frightened. You find yourself thinking about what cancer could mean . . . surgery? Prolonged hospitalization? A totally different life? How would this affect your relationships with family members? And your job? You have a good position and you feel you are valued and respected by colleagues, but what would happen if you had a long absence from work? Your boss is young, would he understand?

With great effort, you force yourself back to more immediate concerns. You call your wife and share the bad news. You spend the rest of the day arranging your work so that you can take a few days off. This is the busy time, and you hate to be gone.

After thinking about it, you decide not to tell anyone at the office about the X-ray until you know for sure what the problem is.

The 10 days drag. You take your medication. As you approach the day
you are to return to see the physician, your wife insists on going with you.

The day finally arrives. Neither you nor your wife feel much like breakfast, but you force down a few bites. You can think of nothing but your problem. You sense that your wife is trying to get your mind off the topic, but conversation is forced and superficial.

You dress in a new sports jacket, one that you had bought for a planned vacation, only to be worn for one of the most depressing trips you have ever taken. You and your wife get in the car and you back out of the driveway. As you drive away from the house, you wonder, "When I come back, will I be the same person?"

When you arrive, you pull into the parking lot, lock the door, and walk through the quiet lot. You feel your anxiety increasing. The steps up to the door seem twice their normal size. Your stomach is in knots, and your palms are sweaty. You tell yourself you're overreacting, but the message doesn't seem to get through.

Out of the corner of your eye you see a beaming mother pushing a baby carriage down the sidewalk, full of enthusiasm and joy for the future – a future which for you seems uncertain.

As you walk down the hallway, you hear your wife comment on remodeling that's been done since she was last here. Her words barely enter your consciousness, as your attention focuses on a patient in a wheel chair. As you continue down the hallway, you pass a couple consoling one another. You find the reception area for your unit. There are several people behind the desk. No one looks up. Finally someone notices you..

Receptionist: "Just fill out this form and put it here in the tray. We'll call you when we're ready."

You complete the form, take a seat, and pick up a magazine. You glance at the cover of the *Newsweek* and realize you read this issue three months ago. Unable to concentrate, you begin to focus on the people in the waiting room, wondering what they're there for. Your wife strikes up a conversation with a middle-aged woman sitting next to you. She asks your wife what she's here for and your wife begins to explain that she's here with you. As the conversation progresses the woman explains that she's here for a blood count because she's on chemotherapy for cancer. You're staring at the woman and all of a sudden you realize how debilitated she looks. You cannot help imagining this to also be your fate. Suddenly you realize the person at the desk is calling your name.

You smile weakly in your wife's direction and walk across the waiting room toward the open door. As you are led to the examining room, the sense of anxiety begins to rise in your chest.

The nurse asks you to step on the scale and then takes your temperature. You comply.

Nurse: "Now let's take your blood pressure. (pause) . . . . It's a little high."

A little high?.... So high that it's a problem you should be worried about? Could this have anything to do with the spot on your lung? You want to ask, but don't for fear of showing your ignorance and your anxiety.

Next she asks a long list of questions about your health history. As you answer the questions, you find your attention is glued to the nurse's face as you try to read her reactions to your answers. Which answers did she think were significant?

Nurse: "Do you have trouble taking medication?"

"I have some difficulty taking pills," you tell her. You notice her eyebrows go up.

Nurse: "How long have you had this difficulty?"

"I've always had difficulty," you respond.

Nurse: "Oh??"

You find yourself fixated on every movement of her face, on every change in the tone of her voice? Is this a problem? Could this have anything to do with the spot on your lungs? What is she thinking?

Nurse: "You didn't eat breakfast today did you?"

You respond, "Yes, no one told me..."

Nurse: "Hmm . . . . We like to have the tests done on an empty stomach."

Tests, what tests? You thought you were simply going to have another X-ray. You explain that you only had coffee and a few bites of toast, and that seemed to satisfy her.

13

The nurse completes her questions and tells you to go to the lab for blood work. You find the lab area, check in at the reception desk, and wait to be called for your tests. After a wait, your name is called and you're led to a room. The next thing you know someone comes in to draw blood. He seems to have difficulty getting the needle into the vein......

Lab Tech: "Boy you really have bad veins here, don't you. I usually don't have any trouble at all."

You wonder what the comment means. Is the person just trying to make small talk? Could your "vein problem" be related to the spot on the lung? You'd like to find a way to ask, but the right words won't come to you.

The lab technician turns to leave, commenting that someone will be with you soon to take you to X-ray. A woman comes and escorts you to the X-ray area. She says nothing – neither do you. After a chest X-ray, you're taken back to the examining room. After a half hour, the X-ray technician appears and says:

"I am going to check the X-rays to be sure they are okay. I'll be back to let you know"

Well, you think to your self, in a few minutes I'll know . . . . The technician returns, and tells you they're okay. "Then there's no spot on the lung?" you ask.

X-Ray Technician: "Oh, I'm afraid I can't tell you about that. All I meant is that the pictures are clear. Your doctor will have to tell you what they show."

You ask if your doctor will be there to see you. The technician replies:

"I really can't tell you. As far as I'm concerned you're done. Check with the nurse to see if they need you for anything else today."

You find your nurse and ask whether you are to take further tests.

Nurse: "No, that's it. Your physician may want further tests, depending on the results of those you've had so far."

"Will I be able to speak with my physician now?" you ask. She asks if you have an appointment with him. "No," you respond, "but..."

Nurse: "Well, I'm sure he's busy now, but you could stop down at his reception area to make an appointment."

As your nurse turns to leave, you ask who will tell you the tests results? She tells you that if the tests are positive your physician will call you. She leaves.

Your mind is spinning. What will the tests show? Did the breakfast you ate interfere with the tests? When will you hear something? You've already waited for ten unbearable days. If you don't hear within a couple of days, should you assume everything's OK? What about the high blood pressure? What will happen next? Hospitalization? More Tests?

You walk back out to the reception area where your wife is waiting. Your eyes meet hers as you pass through the door. You try to force a smile to hide your feelings. She asks how everything went? You struggle in vain to think of something to say as you pick up your coat and walk toward the door.

Understanding the Patient Perspective

Suppose that as the patient referred to above, you received a questionnaire from the health center. Imagine that one of the questions asked you to indicate how satisfied you were with the quality of care you received:

1. Overall, how satisfied were you "very satisfied," "somewhat satisfied," "neutral," "somewhat dissatisfied," or "very dissatisfied" with the care you received?

    __ Very satisfied
    __ Somewhat satisfied
    __ Neutral
    __ Somewhat dissatisfied
    __ Very dissatisfied

2. Why?

3. What thoughts and feelings did you have as the patient?

4. What events stand out in your mind from your visit to the health center as being particularly memorable – either positively or negatively?

5. Based on your experience, do you have an impression of the organization and its staff? What image do you have? On what is the impression based?

6. In what ways were the staff members you encountered helpful?

7. In what ways did the staff members intentionally or unintentionally contribute to your discomfort, confusion, and anxiety?

8. If friends, neighbors, or colleagues asked you about your thoughts about the health center, what would you tell them about this experience?"

9. Looking ahead three to six months, what do you think you'll remember of your experience?

Most people indicate that they would be "somewhat dissatisfied" or "very dissatisfied" if they were the patient in the preceding circumstance. It is interesting to note, however, that no glaring clinical or technical problems occurred in the scenario. For instance, the patient did not receive the wrong medication, nor were incorrect diagnostic tests conducted.

To the extent that we are dissatisfied it is due to a lack of interpersonal sensitivity and information-providing, rather than to clinical or technical inadequacies.

Even for knowledgeable health care professionals, becoming a patient can be a troublesome and difficult experience, one in which caregiver interpersonal sensitivity and skill becomes very important. This is well illustrated in the following passage from *A Leg to Stand On,* written by physician Oliver Sacks (1984, p. 46). In the quotation, Sachs describes his own feelings on becoming hospitalized after sustaining a serious leg injury while mountain climbing:

> " . . . to these grotesque fantasies (of the accident) were added the realities of admission, the systematic depersonalization which goes with becoming-a-patient. One's own clothes are replaced by an anonymous white nightgown, one's wrist is clasped by an identification bracelet with a number. One becomes subject to institutional rules and regulations. One is no longer a free agent . . . one is no longer in the world-at-large. It is strictly analogous to becoming a prisoner, and humiliatingly reminiscent of one's first day at school. . . . One understands that this is protective, but it is quite dreadful too. And I was seized, overwhelmed, by this dread, this elemental sense of dread of degradation, throughout the dragged-out formalities of admission, until – suddenly, wonderfully – humanity broke in, in the first lovely moment I was addressed as myself, and not merely as an "admission" or *thing.*

Adapting to any new situation can be difficult. In the case of health care, all the usual problems of adjusting to a novel situation are magnified due to:

- Loss of control - a patient must depend on others in areas where he or she is used to taking charge.

- Confusion – about the meaning of medical terminology (e.g., plural aspiration, hemotology, OB/GYN, oncology); the significance of various measures (e.g., blood pressure, pulse, etc.); the purpose of tests and procedures (stress tests, EKG); and uncertainty as to what will happen next, who will come in the room next, the patient role, and so on.

- Anxiety about one's physical well-being, family, and/or job.

For many patients, these factors often lead to impaired communication – to an inability to ask the right questions, to listen effectively, or to express oneself fully or considerately. Given this, everything a staff member does and says – every action, expression or gesture – is a message of vital importance to a patient and his or her feelings about the situation, the health care facility, the staff, and his or her own health problem. These messages may reassure and calm, helping the individual overcome change, loss of control, confusion, and anxiety about his or her health. And this in turn can help the individual feel comfortable to ask needed questions and listen effectively. Or, often unintentionally, a staff member may frustrate, frighten, or in other ways contribute to already troubled feelings and distressed communication and information processing.

Insights From Patients

Much can be learned about the nature of relationship quality from patients themselves. Not surprisingly a number of researchers have emphasized the patient perspective in their work (e.g. Bertakis, 1977; Ellmer & Olbrisch, 1983; Greenfield, Kaplan & Ware, 1985, 1986; Kaplan, Greenfield & Ware, 1989; Leebov, 1988; Pascoe, 1983; Ruben, 1985; Ware & Davies, 1983; Waitzkin, 1984, 1986).

One focus of my own patient-centered research over the past several years has been to determine what patients most remember from hospital stays and visits to health centers (Ruben, 1985, 1986, 1987, 1990a, 1990b, 1991, 1992b; Ruben & Bowman, 1986; Ruben, Guttman & Christensen, 1992; Ruben & Ruben, 1988; Ruben, Zakahi & Kreps, 1985). The research involved nearly 4,000 patients at six different hospitals and health services. See "Notes" for details. As a part of the project, patients were asked to:

> "Think back to your stay at the hospital [or visit to the HMO or health center] and describe, in a sentence or two, your most memorable positive or negative experience. (This can be any experience related to the hospital [or HMO or health center], its staff or services)."

Patients' responses were then categorized into one of the following six categories:

"Most memorable experiences related to . . ."

1. Clinical/technical facets of the treatment (abbreviated as: <u>clinical</u>).

2. The institutions policies and procedures (abbreviated as: <u>policies</u>).

3. The institutions facilities/accommodations (abbreviated as: <u>facilities</u>);

4. Aspects of their treatment relating to personal treatment and/or interpersonal communication (abbreviated as: <u>interpersonal</u>).

5. The quality and/or quantity of information provided (abbreviated as: <u>information</u>).

6. Other (abbreviated as: <u>other</u>).

A summary of the findings from these studies is presented in Table 3.1. For each of the health care institutions, the six categories are listed in order based on how frequently they were mentioned in patients' "stories" about what they most remembered. The last column presents an overall ranking of the six categories based on all patient responses at all six health care facilities.

Study Findings

At each of the hospitals or health care facilities studied, patients more frequently recounted experiences involving the quality of their relationships with caregivers – and the way they were treated interpersonally – than circumstances related to all other facets of their experience. Examples of most-remembered events that were classified in this category were: "The friendly attitude makes you feel relaxed when you are tense" and "Many technicians, in my opinion, lacked compassion and concern. They also had no respect for my dignity or modesty. A friendly smile would have helped. They did what they were trained to do and that's all." Table 3.2 lists additional representative responses. Considering patients at all the six health care facilities, interpersonal communication and relationship factors accounted for a remarkable 46.7 percent of all recounted experiences.

At five of the six facilities the "Clinical/Technical" category ranked second; in the case of the ambulatory health care center, the rank was third. Overall, clinical and technical aspects of care – exemplified by statements such as "Got better fast. Identified problem and gave medicine quickly" and "They don't know what they're doing... couldn't find vein" – accounted for only 27.0 percent of all responses.

Health care facilities – which included food in the case of the hospitals – ranked fourth overall, accounting for 7.3 percent of the experiences patients recalled. Examples of responses in this category included: "The ER is very dirty" and "I loved having my own shower in my room." Other examples are provided in Table 3.2.

"Policies and Procedures" accounted for 9.4 percent of the responses overall. Illustrative statements include: "The admissions testing should all be done on one floor" and "Mental patients should not be allowed on floors with other patients."

The "Quality and Quantity of Information Provided" ranked fifth overall at 5.8 percent, including recollections such as: "The night before my operation the doctor explained the operation to me. This relaxed me" and "Doctors should tell patients results of tests and should give more information about patients' illnesses."

The category labelled "other" – which included factors such as cost, convenience, and miscellaneous additional factors – ranked sixth at 3.9 percent. Examples included: "Convenient" and "Would go (to another facility) if I could."

"Personal Treatment/Interpersonal Communication" and "Quality/Quantity of Information Provided" are categorized separately in this study, but it could be argued that they should be combined since both are facets of interpersonal communication. "The quality and quantity of information" category refers to the *content* of communication, while the "interpersonal treatment" aspects refers to the *relationship building* facets of the process. The relationship between "informational aspects" and "personal treatment aspects" of communication in this study parallels the distinction between *content* and *relational* dimensions of interpersonal communication discussed by Watzlawick, Beavin, and Jackson (1966). They note that both aspects of communication are important, and that both may occur simultaneously. If these two categories were combined, the primary role of interpersonal communication in patient recollections of their health care experiences would be emphasized even more dramatically. Together the categories account for 52.5% of reported experiences across the six study sites.

Table 3.1

Factors Associated with Patients' Most Memorable Experiences at Six Health Care Institutions

Rank Order	Acute Care Hospital[1] 582 Bed-Community (N = 204)		Acute Care Hospital[2] 206 Bed-Urban (N = 96)		Acute Care Hospital[3] 248 Bed-Suburban (N = 286)		Acute Care Hospital[4] 354-Bed Community (N = 217)		Rehab Hospital[5] 88 Bed-Regional (N = 94)		Ambulatory Care Center-University[6] 84,867 Visits (N = 228)		Combined Data – Six Institutions (N = 1125)	
	Factor	Percent	Factor	Percent	Factor	Percent	Factor	Percent	Factor	Percent	Factor	Percent	Factor	Percent
First	Interpersonal	39.2%	Interpersonal	47.9%	Interpersonal	46.5%	Interpersonal	58.5%	Interpersonal	56.4%	Interpersonal	37.7%	Interpersonal	46.7%
Second	Clinical	34.8%	Clinical	25.0%	Clinical	33.2%	Clinical	24.9%	Clinical	19.2%	Policies	22.4%	Clinical	27.0%
Third	Information	6.9%	Facilities	12.5%	Information	10.1%	Facilities	6.5%	Facilities	18.1%	Clinical	18.4%	Policies	9.4%
Fourth	Other	6.9%	Policies	9.4%	Policies	5.2%	Policies	6.0%	Policies	5.3%	Information	11.8%	Facilities	7.3%
Fifth	Policies	6.4%	Other	4.2%	Facilities	3.2%	Information	3.7%	Other	1.1%	Other	7.9%	Information	5.8%
Sixth	Facilities	5.9%	Information	1.0	Other	1.8	Other	.5%	Information	0%	Facilities	1.8%	Other	3.9%

[1]Reported in Ruben, 1992b; B. Ruben, Zakahi & Kreps, 1985. [2]Reported in B. Ruben, 1992b; B. Ruben & J. Ruben, 1988. [3]Reported in Ruben, 1990b, 1992b; Ruben & Bowman, 1987; Ruben, 1986. [4]Reported in B. Ruben, 1987, 1992b. [5]Reported in B. Ruben, 1992b; B. Ruben & J. Ruben, 1987. [6]Reported in B. Ruben, 1990b, 1992b; Ruben, Christensen & Guttman, 1990; Ruben, Guttman & Christensen, 1992.

Table 3.2
Patients' Most Memorable Experiences:
Representative Responses

Personal Treatment/Interpersonal Communication

"Many technicians, in my opinion, lacked compassion and concern. They also had no respect for my dignity or modesty. A friendly smile would have helped. They did what they were trained to do and that's all."

"Seeing physician... I was very nervous but she made me feel calm. Made me feel comfortable."

"Please let us feel like we're human."

"The staff gave me the impression that they were interested in me as a person rather than in just doing a job of taking care of me."

"All physicians are nice . . . . They seem to care."

"Without exception, every nurse on the floor took care of my father as if he were their father."

"Nurses discuss each patient openly to other nurses, affording anyone in a nearby room an earful."

"The most pleasant experience was that most of the people treated me very well."

"The guards and the receptionists were very impolite with my family and myself."

"The friendly attitude makes you feel relaxed when you are tense."

Clinical/Technical

"Got better fast. Identified problem and gave medicine quickly."

"A female doctor was looking to give me an intravenous without checking my name or room number. She had wrong room, wrong sex."

"They don't know what they're doing... couldn't find vein."

"I was happy with the services in the Emergency Room. I was admitted and treated quickly."

"Blood test didn't hurt at all."

"The help of the nurses in the maternity ward . . .(they) knew when to help me and when to let me do things on my own."

"I was very unhappy because I had to wait three days for a plastic surgeon for a cut on my lip."

"The RN almost gave my infection medicine to my roommate who was very allergic to it."

"They never X-rayed anything. Just said it was a sprain."

Facilities/Accommodations

"The birthing room facilities were peaceful and beautiful."

"The ER is very dirty."

"Get a nicer waiting area. Chairs are uncomfortable."

"I have gone to college previously in New York State. The health service building here is much better than what I am used to."

"I loved having my own shower in my room."

"Noisy children are unattended and drunken adults bother the patients."

"Smoke from the nurses' lounge was _very_ unpleasant."

Policies/Procedures

"They let you walk in. You don't need an appointment."

"Too much paperwork... too confusing when you first walk in. You don't know where to go or what to do."

"I was impressed by the lack of waiting."

"I was told to come back Monday for a blood test because they don't do blood tests after 12:00. It was very annoying."

"The admissions testing should all be done on one floor."

"Mental patients should not be allowed on floors with other patients."

"Waiting time is too long. Waited two hours for a shot."

Quality/Quantity of Information Provided

"Doctors should tell patients results of tests and they should give more information about patient's illness."

"The night before my operation the doctor explained the operation to me. This relaxed me."

"The emergency room should keep you informed as to why you are lying there for so long."

"The physician explained everything in detail."

"The doctor didn't tell me he was going on vacation, so no one knew who was supposed to take out my stitches."

"A staff member told me how she reduces stress . . . she was friendly."

"When you need to buy a product at the pharmacy, they are never too busy to give you recommendations."

"Wish they could better explain about blood test results."

Other
(General Statements, Convenience, Cost)

"Everything was very nice."

"Would go (to another facility) if I could wait."

"Came away with positive impression."

"Convenient."

Interpreting the Findings:
The Importance of Interpersonal Communication

What do these findings mean? To be sure, these results tell us nothing definitive about how patients were <u>actually</u> cared for. They do, however, tell us a great deal about how patients <u>perceive</u> they were treated, and perhaps more interestingly, about the <u>criteria they use</u> in evaluating the quality of care they receive. By implication, the study also tells us about probable sources of satisfaction and dissatisfaction among patients and helps us understand the basis upon which images of health services are formed.

The findings from this project argue convincingly that patients in a variety of health care settings place a very high premium on personal treatment, interpersonal communication, and relationships in forming their impressions of a health care institution and its staff.

As can be discerned from the sampling of patient responses, the research also indicates that *all staff play a vital role in creating the experiences which are most critical and memorable to patients.* Nurses, nurse practitioners, receptionists, and other staff, as well as physicians, are mentioned in patients' comments. For instance, in the case of the ambulatory care facility (Ruben, 1990; Ruben, Guttman & Christensen, 1990, 1992), nurses and nurse practitioners were most often mentioned. As shown in Table 3.3, they were referred to in 34.3 percent of the narratives on memorable experiences, and generally in a positive context (60.6% positive vs. 39.4% negative). Physicians were mentioned in 29.2 percent of the recounted scenarios (64.3% positive vs. 35.7% negative). Receptionists and other non-technical staff were recalled in 26% of the noted experiences, with a majority (56.0% vs. 44.0%) positive.

Again, it is important to remember that these results refer to patient perceptions. However, it is equally important to remind ourselves of the many reasons why the patient perspective and relationship quality are important. Beyond contributing to a patient's satisfaction or dissatisfaction with health care systems in general, relationship quality affects patient compliance and the course of treatment. It is also the basis for the reputation and image of individual staff members and the health center as an organization, it influences the probability of malpractice litigation, and it facilitates or impedes the appropriate utilization of health care services and facilities.

Insights from Other Settings

This section of the chapter provides a brief summary of two classic and two less familiar behavioral science research studies conducted in very diverse settings. At first glance, studies focused on a factory, classroom, junior college, and pet shop may seem unrelated to health care relationships or even to one another. However, their relevance and implications for bettering our understanding of quality caregiver-patient relationships – and caregiver-caregiver relationships – will become apparent.

Table 3.3
Caregiver Role and Valence of
Most Remembered Experiences

Ranked Roles	No. of Positive Experiences Percent of Experiences	No. of Negative Experiences Percent of Experiences	Total Experiences Percent of All Experiences
Nurses/Nurse Practitioners	20/60.6%	13/39.4%	33/34.3%
Physicians	18/64.3%	10/35.7%	28/29.2%
Receptionist and Other Staff	14/56.0%	11/44.0%	25/26.0%
Lab/Technical Staff	9/90.0%	1/10.0%	10/10.4%
TOTAL	61/63.5%	35/36.5%	96/99.9%

The Factory: "The Western Electric Studies"

What has come to be called "The Hawthorne Effect" was first discovered by F. J. Roethlisberger and William J. Dickson in a two-year study of workers at the Western Electric Company Hawthorne Works in Chicago. Their study was described in detail in Management and the Worker (1941).

The research focused on working conditions, morale, and productivity. Roethlisberger and Dickson set up experimental work rooms and groups to study the impact of such factors as the length of the work day, the length of the work week, and the introduction of breaks during the day. Who would have guessed that what began as a rather routine study would produce results the researchers came to refer to as "astonishing" (Roethlisberger & Dickson, p. 87)?

Much to their surprise, the researchers found that regardless of what specific changes they introduced into the experimental environment – whether they shortened working hours, days and weeks, for instance – worker productivity improved. Every change they made in the subjects' environment seemed to increase productivity. They assumed the finding must somehow be the result of some unrecognized factors in the experimental environment, so they systematically examined the relationship between environmental factors and variations in productivity. Still they found no explanation. By the end of the two-year study, efforts to explain the increased productivity had led to an examination of every imaginable explanation including environmental factors, worker fatigue and monotony, wage incentives, and method of supervision. They went to such levels of detail as to test for the possible impact of temperature, humidity, and even seasonal variation.

After all was said and done, they concluded that differences in productivity were not due to specific changes in the experimental design. Rather, *greater productivity resulted from the positive interpersonal relationships and unusual level of supervisor attention that was present in the experimental group at every phase of the research.* The experiment had fostered closer working relations and had established greater workers' confidence and trust in supervisors than was present in the normal working group situation. Supervisor-worker relations in the experimental room were discovered to have more the flavor of an "office" than a "shop," creating an atmosphere in which workers had become the focus of considerable attention from top management. And indeed it was the increased attention along with productive relationships between workers that had heightened productivity.

The Classroom: Pygmalion in the Classroom

In their book, Pygmalion in the Classroom, Robert Rosenthal and Lenore Jacobson (1968) reported on their research on the impact of teacher expectations on students' intellectual development. They argued persuasively that when teachers expect high or low performances from particular students, their own behavior toward these students is sufficiently different to produce these outcomes through a "self-fulfilling prophecy." That is, if as a teacher I believe John to be a talented child I'll subsequently treat him as if he were, and he will be influenced to become talented by my expectations.

Further studies examined this contention in some depth. Not all studies produced the so-called "pygmalion effect," and controversies developed as to whether these inconsistencies were the result of inappropriate research methods or whether there were underlying problems with the theory.

Despite occasionally inconsistent findings, the weight of evidence supports the original theory: *Teachers' beliefs that particular students are of superior or inferior ability tend to lead to student achievement levels consistent with the expectations.* When teachers' expectations are high, student performances match these expectations; conversely, when teachers have low expectations, lower levels of performance result (Seaver, 1973).

The Junior College: A Study of Adaptation

In 1986, John Herrling, a doctoral candidate in the Rutgers Graduate School of Education undertook a thesis study designed to gain a better understanding of the dynamics of student adaptation to junior colleges. It is well documented in the literature of higher education that attrition rates are very high during the first semester of enrollment; a chief goal of this study was to identify the factors leading to this outcome. Herrling designed a qualitative, ethnographic study in which he met with students at several points during the semester for open-ended, taped conversations about the process of adapting to college. His goal was to gain an in-depth understanding of the dynamics of adaptation and of the attrition process from a student's point of view.

In designing the study, Herrling felt it was important to select a large initial sample of students. Otherwise, if too many students dropped out during the semester, he would be unable to make comparisons between "drop out" and "adapter" groups at the conclusion of the study. Herrling determined that the average first semester attrition rate for the institution where the study was taking place was 30 to 40 percent. He wanted the final sample size to be in the range of 20 students, so he began with a random sample of thirty-two students. He reasoned that even with a 40 percent drop-out rate, he would be left with a study population of 19 or 20 students who would complete the first semester. But Herrling was very surprised by his results. At the end of the first semester, only 3 of the 32 students had left the college – an attrition rate of 9 percent – rather than the usual 30 to 40 percent.

How can this finding be interpreted? Initially, Herrling feared that somehow his initial sample had been a biased one. He carefully considered a variety of possibilities. In reexamining the demographics of his sample, however, he confirmed that the group was representative in terms of high school grades, SAT scores, curriculum studied, and other descriptive characteristics. After much deliberation and careful analysis of the tapes and transcripts from the interviews, he concluded that rather than being an unfortunate circumstance of an unrepresentative sample, the low attrition rate in the study group was instead a truly significant finding in its own right. *Unlike the typical group of college students, this group of 32 students had in effect their own personal counselor – Herrling – who met with them regularly throughout the semester, talked with them, and had a genuine interest in their concerns and in their experiences.*

The Pet Shop: Companionship Boutique

Pet stores sell pets and pet supplies. Nearly every major mall has such stores and they are generally crowded with shoppers cooing and smiling at creatures through the glass and screens. Previously, it was suggested that pet stores sell pets. It may actually be more accurate to say that they sell potential companionship. There are the cute little bunnies, cuddly kittens, exotic fish, high and low verbal birds, and perky puppies. And for the less "warm and fuzzy" types there are snakes, rats and gerbils and cousins of all colors, shapes and sizes.

Much can be learned about quality human relationships from pets, and a fair amount of research has been conducted on pets and the impact of the relationships we have with them. For instance, one study found that introducing pets into the lives of terminal cancer patients (Muschel, 1984) or geriatric patients (Brickel, 1986) had significant positive consequences psychologically and socially. Other studies (Friedmann, Katcher, Lynch & Thomas, 1980) have suggested that pet ownership is a strong predictor of one-year survival among postcoronary patients. Research also shows that older people (65 and over) who are closely attached to a pet are less likely to exhibit symptoms of depression (Garrity, Stallones, Marx & Johnson, 1989). Studies (Garity et. al. 1989; Ory & Goldberg, 1983) have also indicated that individuals with greater attachment to pets have better mental health. In essence, these studies suggest that attachment to or having a significant relationship with a pet may serve the same beneficial role as significant human attachments in times of stress, providing not only a source of companionship but an aid to health and relaxation.

A particularly striking piece of research takes this perspective a bit further to examine whether pet ownership has an effect upon the extent of the use of physician services (Siegel, 1990). Remarkably, the study finds that elderly individuals with pets had fewer contacts with doctors (total doctor contacts and respondent-initiated contacts) than those without pets. Even more remarkably, the study found that individuals with stressful lives and who did not own pets had significantly more doctor contacts than non-pet owners (10.37 contacts per year compared to 8.38).

Are all pet relationships equally effective in this regard? Apparently not. Dogs seem to make better relationship partners than cats or birds. For individuals who did not own a dog, doctor contacts increased as levels of stress increased (10.39 contacts for high stress individuals compared to 8.37 for low stress). However, for dog owners with high and low levels of stress, there was not a significant difference between their total annual number of doctor contacts (Siegel, 1990). This result did not occur for the owners of both cats and birds.

Thus, this study tells us that older people who don't have pets can expect more doctor contacts than individuals with pets. Furthermore, individuals with pets – particularly dogs – are helped by these relationships in times of stress (Siegel, 1990).

There are other insights to be learned from our relationships with pets, dogs in particular – insights about relationships and what makes them work. What is it, exactly, that dogs do for their part in relationships that apparently makes them such ideal partners? Some dogs provide protection. But this is certainly not the case with the majority of pet dogs. Even if they lack the ability to protect their owners, they may still be wonderful companions. Perhaps, the reason dogs are capable of being such great pals is that they exhibit a number of the qualities that are highly valued in human companions. Think about it: Dogs are attentive, interested, trusting, loyal, and tolerant. They are nonargumentative and seem, at times, able to demonstrate compassion and empathy. Some dogs are even masters of good eye contact. Collectively, these are many of the charactertistics we value in friends and companions; such behavior provides a sense of security and reassurance and confirms our sense of worth.

I overheard an interesting and relevant conversation in a shopping mall recently that seemed to capture much of what research on the topic has to say. The topic was dogs:

To your dog it doesn't matter what you look like, whether you've had a good day or or bad one, whether you have performed brilliantly or ineptly that day, how you feel or what you say. You walk in the door and your dog comes running up to you and wags its tail like you're the most important, wonderful person in the world. . . and loves you.

Conclusion

Whether we take our insights from patients, the factory, classroom, junior college, or pet store a common theme emerges. Quality relationships are a valued, valuable and all-too-scarce resource in medical encounters and contemporary life in general. However, this scarcity is not an inevitable circumstance. We each have the power to build and maintain more meaningful, satisfying relationships through a very fundamental communication process that begins with the genuine expression of interest, empathy, concern, and caring for those around us.

Notes

1. Acute Care Hospital (Community): Random sample - 1,000; returns - 253; response rate - 25.3%.

2. Acute Care Hospital (Urban): Random sample - 381; returns - 96; response rate - 25.2%

3. Acute Care Hospital (Community): Random sample - 1,000; returns - 226; response rate - 22.6%

4. Acute Care Hospital (Suburban): Random sample 927; returns - 338; response rate - 36.5%

5. Rehab Hospital (Regional): Total patient population was surveyed - 360; returns - 130; response rate - 36.1%.

6. Ambulatory Care Center (University) - random point of departure interviewer-aided surveys at three sites - 200; returns - 200; response rate - 100%.

Chapter 4

CAREGIVER-PATIENT COMMUNICATION

"I became all of a sudden desolate and deserted, and felt . . . the essential aloneness of the patient. . . . Desperately now, I wanted communication, and reassurance."
Oliver Sacks, M.D., *"A Leg to Stand On"*

An Overview of the Interpersonal Communication Process

At the heart of the linkage between communication and health care is the interpersonal communication between caregivers and patients and the nature of the relationship which develops as a consequence. Unfortunately, caregiver-patient communication and relationships are as problematic as they are important, embodying all the complexity and challenge – and even greater stress – than are present in most other professional encounters.

In the most basic terms, interpersonal communication is a process of sending and receiving messages in an effort to coordinate meaning. Influencing what would seem to be a very simple process are a number of factors, which include the people, the messages they create, the channels through which messages are exchanged, and the situations in which the exchange takes place.

The process of health communication is an activity which involves four elements: a *sender, messages,* a *channel* and a *receiver,* as shown in Figure 4.1. As suggested in the model a *sender* is a person who creates and transmits a message. The *receiver* is a person who notices and reacts to the message. A *channel* is the means by which *messages* are sent.

In an ongoing conversation between a caregiver and a patient, each is alternately sender and receiver. A caregiver serves as a sender when he or she asks "Hello, how are you?" The patient to whom the caregiver is speaking is the receiver. When the patient responds, "Fine, how are you?" he or she becomes the sender, and the caregiver assumes the role of receiver, and so on. This descriptions makes communication sound quite simple, but it is actually quite complex for reasons we will discuss in the following sections.

29

Figure 4.1
The Communication Process

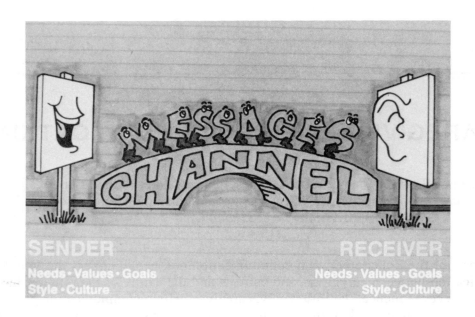

A Number of Factors Affect the Sender and Receiver.

In any situation, a sender and receiver have their own unique needs, values, attitudes, styles, education, and cultural backgrounds which they bring with them to the communication situation. All of these characteristics affect the individuals and what transpires between them. As we will discuss shortly, differences between caregivers and patients are often substantial and create formidable impediments to communication.

Communication Involves Both Verbal and Nonverbal Messages.

Most people think of "talking" or "writing" when they hear the word "communication." Obviously, talking – and to a lesser extent writing – is a critical component of caregiver-patient communication. However, there are also a number of *non-verbal* aspects of caregiver-patient communication, that include gestures, posture, eye behavior, actions, touch, and facial expressions. Anything a caregiver does or fails to do do, says or does not say, can be a message that has an impact on patients, visitors, family, and other staff. See Figure 4.2.

Communication Involves Unintentional as well as Intentional Message Sending.

Many of the messages we send are *intentional,* as when someone asks "Hi, how are you?" Most of the messages we send out, however, are *unintentional* or *accidental,* as

Figure 4.2

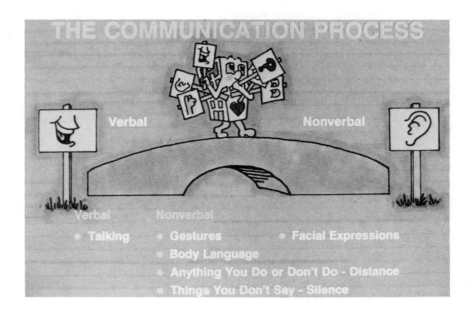

shown in Figure 4.3. The often-unconscious way we say something, the looks on our faces, our gestures, even the words we choose when we're not concentrating on communication are all potentially important messages to receivers.

Communication Involves Receiving Messages as Well as Sending Them.

Adding complexity to the health communication process is the fact that caregivers must serve as information receivers as well as senders. See Figure 4.4. While most people spend much less time worrying about their role as an information receiver, message-receiving skills are often more important and difficult than message-sending skills.

As a receiver, three processes are involved:

• Listening

• Observing

• Interpreting

It is through sensitive message reception – listening, interpreting, and observing – that we gain insight into others' thoughts, concerns, fears, and unspoken questions. It's also through receiving that we get information necessary to make informed decisions about what messages to send and when and how to send them.

31

Figure 4.3

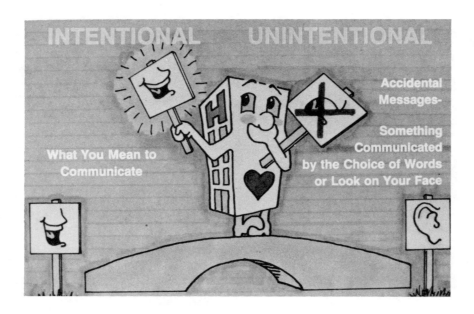

Health Communication Involves Repetitive Activities

Another factor that adds to the complexity of the health situation is repetition. In most health care roles, caregivers deal with similar situations day-in and day-out. For the physician, transporter, X-ray technician, or receptionist, it is easy to become mechanical as a sender and receiver in such a situation. What is "routine" for a caregiver it is likely to be a "crisis" for the patient, and special effort is required to approach each situation and person as unique.

Interpersonal Communication Involves Both Content and Relationships

When people talk to one another their messages convey content about a topic as well as information that shapes the tone or climate of the relationship between the individuals. There are many ways to get an idea or thought across. While any of these may have essentially the same content, messages may differ greatly from one another in terms of whether they are warm or cold, encouraging or discouraging, friendly or unfriendly, or critical or supportive. Particularly in stressful or repetitive communication situations, caregivers may inadvertently concentrate on the content component of interpersonal communication, while overlooking or neglecting equally-important relationship building aspects of conversation.

Figure 4.4

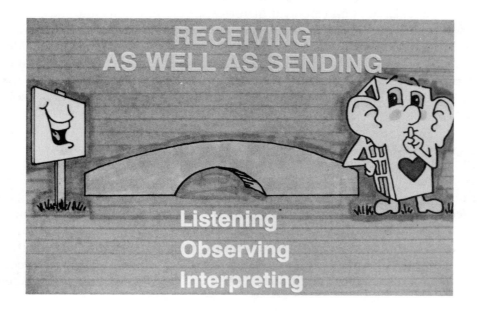

RECEIVING
AS WELL AS SENDING

Listening
Observing
Interpreting

Interpersonal Communication and Relationships

Communication works efficiently and effectively in relationships where there are compatibilities between sender and receiver in terms of needs, priorities, styles, culture, and perspective. When incompatibilities of various kinds exist, interpersonal communication and the development of relationships are a much greater challenge. Caregiver-patient communication is perhaps the prototypical example of this circumstance. One reason has to do with differences in needs the individuals bring to the situation. Caregivers bring particular needs to their encounters with patients, including the desire for an accurate medical history, information pertinent to diagnosis of the presenting problem, efficient information exchange and patient compliance and cooperation. For their part, patients enter the situation with needs that only partially correspond to those of the physician, including not only clinical care but also information, explanation, attention, empathy, and reassurance.

Barriers to Relationship Quality

As with the teacher and student, the attorney and client, or the librarian and the information seeker, the relationship between the caregiver and the patient is *asymmetrical* because expertise and power are unevenly distributed. While both parties to such relationships can be said to have a common purpose, they seldom share common perspectives.

Physicians, nurses, lab technicians, receptionists, administrators, and other staff come to encounters as knowledgeable professionals, at home in the environment in which the interactions are occurring, seeing patients on a schedule which they set. Factors such as time

33

pressures, job stress, the burden of paperwork, threat of malpractice, difficult patients, interpersonal stress, and problems of coordination and repetition present barriers for the caregiver. Nonetheless, caregivers are familiar with terminology and protocols, comfortable with the tasks at hand (medical histories, physical exams and diagnostic procedures), and generally equipped with substantial experience with respect to the range of medical problems and circumstances that present themselves. Health care providers make their judgments of the quality of care using clinical and technical criteria: Have correct diagnostic procedures been followed? Were appropriate treatment protocols adhered to? Was testing conducted in a technically correct manner? (Droste, 1988; Siegel, 1986; 1990; Steiber, 1988)

In contrast, patients come to the relationship looking for help in some form. They do so in an environment that is unfamiliar and which they may perceive as intimidating. Patients must schedule the encounter at the convenience of the caregivers and often have to wait to be seen. Frequently they enter the interaction anxious about their health, and lacking medical knowledge or relevant professional expertise. For the patient, even routine history-taking, physical exams, and tests are often uncomfortable because they call for levels of verbal disclosure and physical contact normally reserved for intimate relationships. Depending upon the outcome of these encounters, patients may be faced with recommendations for behavioral change, additional testing, or continuing uncertainty about their health status.

To help overcome some of the obstacles to communication, Brown & Morley (1988, p. 144) offer the following suggestions to caregivers:

- Don't hurry; make the patient feel he or she is the only one you have to think about at that moment.

- Greet patients with a comment such as "It's good to see you," rather than "Why are you here today?"

- When possible initiate the contact with patients when they are dressed.

- Communicate with the patient on physicially equal terms. Whenever possible, avoid "talking-down" to a patient while you are standing and he or she is seated and reclining.

- Give patients an opportunity to express their concerns by asking questions like, "Is there anything you're concerned about?"

- Don't interrupt an encounter with a phone call or side conversation unless it is absolutely necessary.

- End each encounter with a personal comment such as "It was good to see you" or "Take care."

- Provide oral and written instructions and information whenever possible.

- Listen carefully to patients, paying particular attention to nonverbal messages.

Chapter 5

THE ANATOMY OF PHYSICIAN-PATIENT COMMUNICATION

"The doctors ... were, I presume, (among the) finest. I vaguely remember them as competent, but in a child's mind doctors represent more than competence; they represent assurance of survival by special people uniquely interested in life."
Irving Louis Horowitz, *Daydreams and Nightmares*

Patients are not alone in their concerns. Physicians are also struggling to cope with the challenges of health care in the 1990s. The following comments from a *Time* cover story, "Sick and Tired: Uneasy Patients May Be Surprised to Find Their Doctors Are Worried Too," underscore some dimensions of the problem (Gibbs, 1989):

"Once most people treated me as a friend and a confidant. These days the malpractice threat has created a definite wedge between a physician and some of his (or her) patients."
Boyd McCracken, Sr., family practitioner, Greenville, IL.

"I think patients have become consumers. They are no longer interested in their doctor, who has perhaps been their doctor for five, six, ten years. They are really interested in what it's going to cost them. It's just like they're going shopping at the local supermarket."
Robert Rogers, ophthalmologist, Pompano Beach, FL.

"Technologies have put a kind of emotional moat between doctor and patient."
David Rogers, Prof. of Medicine, Cornell University Medical College.

"You have to be tolerant. You have to be able to answer questions, and it's got to be an answer that the patient is able to understand. Twenty years ago, I imagine, less explanation would have been necessary."
Jay Alexander, cardiologist, Lake Forest, IL

"(Patients) want the knowledge and precision of the most advanced science, and the care and concern of the old-fashioned practitioner."
Lester King, physician and medical historian, Chicago, IL

"I get no sense they trust me. You tell them, 'You're O.K.' They say, 'No, I'm not O.K. I think I have a brain tumor.' They keep asking, 'How do you really know?'"
Jonathan Licht, neurologist, San Diego, CA

In many ways this situation is quite ironic: "Never have doctors been able to do so much for their patients, and rarely have patients seemed so ungrateful" (Gibbs, 1989, p. 48). Not surprisingly, the lack of gratitude is accompanied by troubling levels of dissatisfaction among patients, as indicated in Table 5.1.

In addition to concerns related directly to patient care, physicians wrestle with administrative and business concerns associated with changing economics of their field. There are also precautions and procedures linked to malpractice considerations, and responsibilities associated with the management and coordination of professional and support staff. And, in addition, there is the substantial commitment of time and energy necessary to keep current with scientific, technological, and clinical advances. As Gibbs (1989) asserts:

... it is simply harder to be a doctor now than it was a generation ago: harder to master the art of the craft, harder to practice, harder to savor the nature pleasures of healing. (p. 48)

Doctors lose the sense of satisfaction that comes from having a personal relationship with patients and helping them through crises, since hospital stays are shorter, patients are sicker, and treatment time is more rushed. (p. 51)

Why Communication and Quality Patient Relations Are Vital for Physicians

In light of the many challenges facing the physician, achieving and maintaining quality in communication and relationships with patients is extremely important. Communication has an impact on patients' outlooks, knowledge levels, attitudes, and behaviors all of which can be very positive influences.

1. Patients As Consumers

More than ever before, health care has become a business. It is a business to hospital, HMO, clinic, and insurance company administrators, and to physicians and other practitioners building a practice. Each increasingly worries about product lines and mix, expense-to-revenue ratios, unionization, cash flow, relations with third party payors, patient satisfaction, and repeat and referral business. Health care is also increasingly a business to patients who bring their expectations as consumers from other settings with them to health care contexts (Haug & Lavin, 1983; President's Commission, 1982).

Table 5.1
Satisfaction and Dissatisfaction with Physicians

In general, do you think doctors do a:	Good job	Poor job
Keeping up with latest medical knowledge	72%	17%
Providing high quality medical care	61%	25%
Diagnosing patients correctly	54%	32%
Being caring with patients	54%	32%
Listening to what patients tell them	46%	45%
Explaining to patients what they are doing	45%	45%
Being on time for appointments	37%	56%
Being fair in the prices charged	22%	70%

(Source: Nancy Gibbs, "Sick and Tired: Uneasy Patients May Be Surprised to Find Their Doctors Are Worried Too," *Time,* July 31, 1989, p. 50. Based on a study conducted by Yankelovich Clancy Shulman, April 4-5, 1989, for Time/CNN Sampling error ± 3%.)

Consumers have come to expect certain kinds of treatment at restaurants, department stores, hotels, and airlines. Most consumers are very well aware of what they regard as their rights, and many are quick to point them out when they are abridged. When dissatisfied with services rendered at a dry cleaner, restaurant, or auto repair shop many people have a well-rehearsed repertoire of responses they can call forth to deal with the situation. While physicians and other medical professionals may not see health care settings as analogous to restaurants or the hotels, a growing number of patients do. So significant is the impact of the trend toward active consumerism, that one writer concludes:

> Physicians certainly cannot hope to satisfy patients who, instructed by the consumer movement, have come to view medicine as a commodity like any other, despite the fact that it is unlike any other. Once people would no more price shop for a doctor than they would for a church. (Gibbs, 1989, p. 50)

While the challenges presented by increasingly demanding consumers are substantial, a commitment to quality interpersonal communication and relationships does a great deal to increase consumer satisfaction and to respond meaningfully to dissatisfaction when it occurs.

2. Perception of Physician Clinical/Technical Competence

Most patients cannot assess clinical and technical competence directly, as noted previously. They do make judgments, however. Often, in these judgments a "halo effect" operates such that impressions of a caregiver's positive or negative attributes "spill over" to lend a positive or negative aura to other actions. In effect, patients unknowingly lose sight of the distinction between clinical competence and communication competence in their evaluations. In the absence of an ability to make clinically-based determinations "the good physician" is often the one who has acquired and effectively employs interpersonal communication strategies and sensitivities.

Physicians are often troubled by the suggestion that patients often do not differentiate between clinical and communication skills, often leading some to pose the following question: "If as a patient you could chose between one of the best clinicians in the country who is rude and inconsiderate" or "a mediocre physician clinically with good interpersonal skills" which would you prefer?

Such a reaction is certainly understandable given the considerable investment doctors make to acquire and maintain clinical competence, and a number of important issues are raised by this question. Certainly if faced with this choice most patients would have little trouble deciding in favor of clinical competence. However, the question makes several assumptions. First, it implies that patients would, in fact, know which physician was clinically superior and which was mediocre; unfortunately, the underlying problem is that few patients can make such a determination. Second, there is the implication that clinical competence and interpersonal competence are mutually-exclusive, and that patients should be forced to choose between a physician who is clinically competent and one who is communicationally competent. Certainly there is no reason to suppose that such a choice is desirable or necessary. Third, the question implies an independence between the physical/clinical on the one hand and the communicational/emotional on the other, which is fundamentally disputed by many scientists and practitioners.

3. Practice Building and Maintenance

Interpersonal communication skill and sensitivity are also essential to creating and sustaining a strong practice. A physician, dentist, or pharmacist who is well-liked by patients becomes the focal point of stories that are told and retold leading to repeat and referral business within a neighborhood or community. Dissatisfaction also has an impact.

38

In *Marketing Strategies for Physicians,* Brown & Morley (1986, p. 61) summarize research identifying reasons why customers are lost:

- Staff discourtesy – 68%

- Product dissatisfaction - 16%

- Competitive Inroads - 11%

- Customers move - 4%

- Customers die - 1%

Brown & Morley (1986, p. 171) note: "Most consumers don't stop buying your product because they've found something better. Rather, they stop because of their experiences with you." In the case of health care "the product" is something much larger than quality clinical care. Consistent with previous discussions, the authors (1986, p. 171) cite a number of other factors of importance to health care consumer satisfaction, most of which relate to interpersonal communication and relationship quality:

- The staff's handling of patients.

- The staff's attitude toward patients.

- The physician's attitude toward patients.

- The time patients must wait to see a physician.

- The time a physician spends with patients.

- The completeness of the service.

- The overall physical environment.

4. Image of Health Care Organization

Probably all practitioners can relate stories of colleagues with booming medical or dental practices whom they would never recommend to a friend or associate. How is it that such physicians achieve such a favorable image and attain such popularity for their practice? As with the reputation of an individual physician, the image of a hospital, HMO, clinic, medical, or dental practice is greatly affected by staff interpersonal skill and sensitivity. Recall research indicating that staff discourtesy alone, accounts for 68% of lost customers (Brown & Morley, 1986, p. 61).

5. Impact on Litigation

Lawyers and health scholars with experience in the area of medical litigation indicate that communication problems of one kind or another are at the root of the great majority of malpractice suits. Plaintiff attorneys report that 70-80 percent of the patients seeking legal assistance to file a malpractice claim do so because they are angry, not just about an adverse medical outcome, but because of breakdowns in communication, failures of physicians or clinic staff to provide information, long waits, and other factors leading to a perception of lack of care, concern, and respect for the patient (Sanders, 1990). The role of communication and relationship quality in medical malpractice is explained as follows in the U.S. Department of Health, Education and Welfare report:

> The quality of the relationship between the patient on one hand and the doctor . . . on the other hand may stimulate the patient either toward or away from filing a malpractice suit. In plain truth, the suit itself is merely tangible proof of the final breakdown in that relationship (HEW, 1973, p. 67).

Sanders (1990) offers a number of specific suggestions in this regard: patients must clearly understand what their hospital, HMO, or clinic experience will involve. When they don't, the result is often misunderstanding, anger, and frustration. All staff must also be made aware of the importance of maintaining the confidentiality of patient information. Patients arriving for an appointment should not be asked their reason for a visit within hearing range of other patients. Billing and insurance matters should always be discussed in a private setting, and conversations regarding patients must never take place in a setting where the discussion can be overheard by others.

Simply stated, available evidence strongly suggests that the probability of a patient initiating litigation is greatly reduced when a physician is interpersonally skilled and sensitive, careful in his or her information providing and handling, and genuinely concerned about creating and maintaining a positive relationship with a patient and/or the family.

6. Influence on Other Staff

Physicians' attitudes and behaviors set the tone for an entire hospital, HMO, care center, or group practice. Actual behaviors are far more impactful than verbalized philosophy, instructions, or statements of intent; in this circumstance as in so many other, actions do speak louder than words. Physicians' communication sensitivity and skill are necessary ingredients to the creation of a positive communication climate between staff and patients, and among members of the health care team.

7. Impact on Health Care

Listed last, but certainly not of least significance is the role of physician-patient communication and relationships relative to health care quality. A growing number of claims suggest the importance of the linkage between communicational/psychological/emotional well-being on the one hand, and physical health on the other. The literature includes work which is philosophical, theoretical, empirical, anecdotal, and testimonial. This is an extensive and fascinating body of literature, one that merits thoughtful consideration.

In this context, however, it is important to comment briefly on two areas of study linking communication to health care. The first are clinical studies Kaplan, Greenfield, and Ware (e.g. 1989; Greenfield, Kaplan & Ware, 1985; 1986), which examine the relationship between physician-patient communication behaviors and health outcomes. The researchers begin by systematically observing and recording specific communication behaviors observed during physician-patient encounters. Three of the dimensions involved are:

1. Patient Effectiveness – Patients' effectiveness in information seeking. (Measurement of factual statements made by the physician compared to the sum of controlling statements made by patients).

2. Interaction Ratio – Patients' involvement in interaction. (Measurement of patients' conversational behaviors compared to physician conversational behaviors).

3. Emotion-Opinion Sharing – The level of emotion and opinion-sharing. (Measurement of emotional expressions and non-factual opinion statements made by physician and patient during the encounter).

Kaplan, Greenfield, and Ware (1989) examine the relationship between these communication measures of health status. Health status was measured physiologically (blood pressure or blood sugar levels), behaviorally (functional status), and subjectively (patient evaluations of overall health status) were consistently related to specific aspects of physician-patient communication. As shown in Table 5.2, physician-patient communication patterns are found to be consistently predictive of health status.

41

Table 5.2
Relationship of Physician-Patient Communication
to Health Status[1]

Measures of Health	Doctor-Patient Communication Indicators		
	Patient Effectiveness Index[2]	Interaction Ratio[3]	Emotion-Opinion Sharing[4]
Subjective			
Self-Rated Overall Health[5]	.42*	.21*	.22*
Behavioral			
Days Lost from Work[6]	-.16	-.30*	-.29*
Number of Health Problems[7]	-.31*	.13	.12
Functional Limitations[8]	-.47*	-.36*	-.46*
Physiological			
Blood Glucose[9]	-.43*	-.29*	-.26*
Blood Pressure[10]	-.36*	-.41*	-.39*

* $P < .05$
1. Pearson Product Moment Correlations
2. Ratio of factual statements by physicians to controlling behaviors by patients
3. Ratio of patient to physician conversational behaviors
4. Total of emotions and and non-factual opinions expressed by physicians and patients
5. "How would you rate your overall health?" (1-4 rating)
6. Total days off from work in previous month.
7. What health problems do you now have?" (sum of problems listed)
8. Physical, social, mobility limitations, e.g. "Are you unable to drive ... ?" (mobility). (Sum of yes responses)
9. Level of glycosylated hemoglobin measured using boronate affinity column kit (range = 6-15).
10. Level of diastolic pressure; average of three consecutive seated readings (range = 60-125).

(Source: S. H. Kaplan, S. Greenfield & J. E. Ware, "Assessing the Effects of Physician-Patient Interactions on the Outcomes of Chronic Disease," *Medical Care,* March 1989, 27(3), *Supplement.*)

Patient Compliance and Non-Compliance

Communication is also important in patient compliance and noncompliance. When problems of noncompliance occur – and unfortunately, this is often – communication patterns of the physician, the patient, or the relationship have usually played a significant role .

Potential Physician Contributions to Non-Compliance:

• Inadequacies in information transmission (e.g. Korsch & Gozzi, 1968; Greenfield, Kaplan & Ware, 1985; Greenfield, Kaplan & Ware, 1986; Korsch & Negrete, 1972; Ruben, 1989; Wertz, Sorenson & Hereen, 1988; Tuckett, et. al., 1985; Waitzkin, 1985; Meichenbaum & Turk, 1987)

   Excess technical/medical language

   Incomplete explanation (diagnosis, rationale)

   Failure to personalize recommendations

   Failure to encourage patient questioning

   Failure to solicit patient commitment

• Inadequacies in information reception (Korsch & Gozzi, 1968; Korsch & Negrete, 1972; Wertz, Sorenson & Hereen, 1988; Ruben, 1992a; Tuckett, et. al., 1985; Ley, 1983)

   Failure to identify patient concerns

   Failure to identify patient reaction/resistance to recommendations

• Inadequacies in interpersonal/social-psychological competence (Cline, 1983; Cline & Cardosi, 1983; Korsch & Negrete, 1972; Ruben, 1989; Siegel, 1986; Thompson, 1986)

   Failure to be sensitive to patient perspective

   Failure to establish rapport

   Lack of displayed respect and empathy

   Failure to build trust

   Failure to build credibility (demonstrated clinical competency relative to case)

Potential Patient Contributions to Non-Compliance:

•Inadequacies in information transmission (Wertz, Sorenson & Hereen, 1988; Waitzkin, 1985; Meichenbaum & Turk, 1987)

>   Failure to provide clear explanation of concerns

>   Incomplete explanation (symptoms, concerns relative to recommendations)

>   Failure to ask questions

• Inadequacies in information reception (Ley, 1983; Ruben, 1992a)

>   Selective attention/perception and distortion

>   Information overload

• Inadequacies in interpersonal/social-psychological competence (Kaplan, Ware & Greenfield, 1986; Korsch & Negrete, 1972; Northouse & Northouse, 1985; Ruben, 1988 Ch 7; 1989; Siegel, 1986; Meichenbaum & Turk, 1987; Thompson, 1986)

>   Denial (of problem, appropriateness of recommendations)

>   Anxiety

>   Dysfunctional attitude toward authority

>   Shyness/reticence/communication apprehension

>   Failure to establish rapport

>   Lack of receptivity to information

Potential Relationship Contributions to Non-Compliance:

• Inadequacies in information exchange (e.g. Korsch & Gozzi, 1968; Greenfield, Kaplan & Ware, 1985; Greenfield, Kaplan & Ware, 1986; Korsch & Negrete, 1972; Ruben, 1989; Wertz, Sorenson & Hereen, 1988; Tuckett, et. al., 1985; Waitzkin, 1985; Thompson, 1986)

>   Inadequate interaction management

• Lack of relationship (e.g. Stewart & Roter, 1989; Thompson, 1986; Pendleton, et. al. 1984; Kleinman, 1980)

>   Failure to negotiate perspectives, concerns

>   Inadequate rapport, trust, respect

• Lack of continuity of relationship

Physician-Patient Encounters

The role of communication can be better understood if one dissects the physician-patient encounters in order to identify its basic structure. The physician-patient encounter involves a series of interpersonal contacts with the physician and other staff members which collectively define the health care experience:

- Pre-visit contact – face-to-face or phone

- Initial contact with staff upon arrival

- Contact with staff in the reception area

- Contact with staff in the examining area

- Contact with staff in lab or X-ray

- Contact with the physician

- Contact with staff when departing

- Post-visit contact with staff or physician – face-to-face, mail, or telephone

The complexity of this encounter is underscored when we consider the process patients go through in deciding to seek health care in the first place. Mechanic (1978, 268-269) finds that decisions as to whether or not to seek health care are based on ten factors:

1. Visibility and recognition of symptoms

2. Extent to which symptoms are perceived as dangerous

3. Extent to which symptoms disrupt family, work, or other social activities

4. Frequency and persistence of symptoms

5. Tolerance for the symptoms

6. Available information, knowledge, and culture assumptions

7. Basic needs that lead to denial

8. Other needs competing with illness response

9. Competing interpretations that can be given to the symptoms once recognized

10. Availability and proximity of treatment resources, and psychological and financial costs.

Motivated by a constellation of these factors, the patient initiates the contact that eventually places him or her in a face-to-face contact with health care staff and a physician. A number of goals guide the encounter once initiated. As shown in Table 5.3, these include

Table 5.3
Objectives of Physician-Patient Encounters

1. To determine the reasons for the patient's visit
    - nature and history of the problem(s)
    - etiology
    - patient's ideas, concerns, and expectations
    - effects of the problem

2. To consider other health problems
    - continuing problems
    - risk factors

3. To select an appropriate action for each problem.

4. To achieve a shared understanding of the problems with the patient.

5. To involve the patient in management of the problems and encourage him/her to accept appropriate responsibility.

6. To use time and resources effectively.

7. To establish or maintain a relationship with the patient which helps to achieve these objectives.

(Source: Based on D. A. Pendleton, T. Schofield, P. Tate, and P. Havelock, *The Consultation: An Approach to Learning and Teaching.* Oxford: Oxford University Press, 1984.)

determining the reasons for the patient's visit, considering other pertinent problems, selecting an appropriate action, achieving a shared understanding of the problems, involving the patient as appropriate in problem solving, utilizing time and resources effectively, and achieving a relationship with the patient which will facilitate achieving these goals.

Interpersonal communication skill and sensitivity is essential to five of the seven listed goals. The exceptions are 3 and 6. In the case of Objective 3, selecting an appropriate action, interpersonal communication may be involved to the extent that conferral with or referral to colleagues takes place.

It has been argued that the efficiency of operation is greatly sacrificed when one places additional emphasis on interpersonal communication. While there may be instances where this is the case, the reverse argument can also be compelling: 1) Many patient-oriented communication behaviors require very little time; 2) effective communication is essential to achieving other goals; 3) small additional quantities time and effort invested "along the way" often eliminate major problems requiring greater expenditures of time and energy if left unaddressed. A modest investment of time on interpersonal communication during various encounters with a particular patient, for instance, often goes a long way toward preventing the more time- and resource- intensive problems of non-compliance, damaged reputation within a community, or malpractice litigation.

Physician-Patient Communication: Barriers and Breakdowns

There are a number of factors affecting physicians that conspire to make physician-patient communication extremely complex and difficult undertaking, among them:

- Time shortages

- Job stress

- The burden of paperwork

- Delays in clinical reports

- Threat of malpractice litigation

- Difficult patients and problems

- Interpersonal stress with colleagues and associates

- Problems of staff coordination

- Monotony of repetitive communication situations

For their part, patients also come to communication encounters with their physicians burdened by various factors, among them:

- Difficulty gaining access

- Confusion about tests, terminology, and procedures

- Anxiety about their health and the encounter situation

- Lack of medical knowledge

- Attitude of professional mystique

- Problems of continuity and coordination among caregivers

- Loss of control

- Ambiguity and confusion regarding to their role as patient

Physicians and patients also come to the encounter with somewhat different needs. Primary needs for the physician are history taking, diagnosis, and treatment with a concern for efficiency. For patients, diagnosis and treatment are important, of course, but so are explanation, empathy, reassurance, and consolation in many instances. Not surprisingly, given the difficulty of health communication in general, and the additional impediments operating in physician-patient encounters, misunderstanding is common and opportunities for facilitating relationships are often missed, as shown in Table 5.4.

Misunderstandings may have a variety of causes, among them insufficient information provided, the use of technical or ambiguous language, and an exclusive reliance on oral communication. For the physician who brings medical knowledge and experience to patient encounters it is easy to assume that an explanation given to a patient is clear and intelligible. However, for the patient who lacks knowledge, experience, medical education, and who may well be anxious about his or her health and the encounter situation, the intended messages may be easily missed, misunderstood, or distorted.

Sugarman and Butters (1985) document some of the communication problems that result from the use of specialized language and technical jargon. Examples of common mala-propisms, where patients were found to confuse the pronunciation of standard medical terminology, include:

- Bleech baby – Breech baby

- Cadillacs – cataracts

- Chicken pops – Chicken Pox

- Coronary seclusion – Coronary occlusion

- Corpse suckles – Red blood corpuscles

- Ferocious (roaches) of the liver – Cirrhosis of the liver

- Hemogoblins – hemoglobin

- Mercy clinic – Emergency clinic

- Monogram – Myelogram

- Sick as hell – Sickle cell anemia

The tendency to rely on oral communication in physician-patient communication, and the problems that result, is worthy of additional discussion. Patients are often anxious during encounters with physicians and lack familiarity with medical terms and not uncommonly, physicians are rushed. To rely solely on oral communication in such a circumstance is to invite incompleteness and error in the communication process. Supplementing oral communication with written communication – notes taken by a patient or written for him or her by the physician – can do much to circumvent these difficulties.

Often, too, patient communication initiatives are inadvertently overlooked or discouraged. Sometimes, physicians simply overlook the cues – which may be indirect or subtle – that indicate a patient has further questions or needs additional clarification. Physicians may assume that patients who have questions will ask them; the absence of overt communication initiatives by the patient is often incorrectly taken as evidence that communication has been clear and effective. I am reminded of the comments of a physician at a seminar who remarked that he had never had a communication problem with a patient in his many years of practice. The evidence for this claim was that patients never had any questions when he was done explaining the situation. It is, of course, possible that this physician is a truly gifted communicator. A more likely explanation, however, is that he has simply been unaware of patients' unmet communication needs, and inadvertently discouraged their communication initiatives. In some more extreme cases, discouragement may be quite overt as in the following recorded exchange:

> Patient: "Doctor, I wanted to ask you a question about what you said before about my diet. . . "
>
> Physician: "Weren't you listening? I just went over all of that."

Other communication results from inadequacies in interaction management. *Interaction management* refers to "turn-taking" in conversations. At one extreme a physician may monopolize the conversation, or on the other extreme he or she may be unresponsive or very abrupt in reacting to patients' communication initiatives.

Studies of physician-patient encounters by Waitzkin (1985, 1991) determined that when physicians and their patients were asked how much patients wanted to know, doctors incorrectly underestimated their patient's information needs in two out of three encounters. He also found that while physicians estimated that they spend about 12 minutes giving information to patients, they actually spent an average of 1.3 minutes giving information. Physicians in the study underestimated how much their patients want to know two-thirds of the time. They also estimated that they spend about nine times as long informing patients as they actually did. Appointments averaged 10-15 minutes, with most of the time devoted to physical examinations. Waitzkin indicated that physicians who earn less spent more time with patients, while more highly-paid doctors saw more patients per day. Research also indicated that women got slightly more time and information than men. These differences could be attributed to women asking more questions and insisting on more verbal

Table 5.5
Common Physician-Patient Communication Outcomes

- Misunderstanding

    Insufficient information given

    Use of technical or ambiguous language

    Exclusive reliance on oral communication

- Patient Communication is Discouraged

    Patients' attempts to communicate overlooked

    Interaction management inadequacies:

        Monopolizing time available for communication; or
        Unresponsiveness to patient communication initiatives

    Reliance on closed-ended questions

    Patients' concerns ignored or minimized

    Patients' statements or questions dismissed or ignored

    Departure or tasks undertaken while a patient is speaking.

- Missed Opportunities to Establish Rapport

    Inadequate greetings and closings

    Use of impersonal language

    Lack of reference to medical record

    Minimal eye contact and inadequacies in other aspects of nonverbal communication

interaction, leading Waitzkin to conclude that patients are going to have to be assertive to get questions answered.

Physician' reliance on *closed-end questions* – questions to which a patient can simply answer "yes" or "no" – is another reason for a lack of information exchange between physician and patient. Closed-end questions, such as "Do you have any questions," do less to encourage patient communication initiatives, than *open-ended questions?* such as "What questions do you have?" which encourage the patient to articulate their questions or concerns. The wording of open-ended questions can also be important, as Frankel and Beckman (1989) explain. Patients who were asked "What worries you about this problem?" responded that they were not worried. However, when the same patients were asked "What concerns you about the problem?" more than one-third voiced concerns.

Communication is also discouraged when patient concerns are ignored or minimized. This takes place when a patient's questions or statements are not responded to or when the significance or relevance of a patient concern or question is minimized intentionally or unintentionally by a physician. This occurs when a patient is told that information he or she is volunteering "isn't important" or "is not relevant." The physician's intention, of course, is to indicate that the information isn't necessary to the problem at hand. However, the fact that the patient has chosen to volunteer the information suggests that he or she does see it is pertinent. Being told that one's comments are not important or irrelevant is likely to be interpreted to mean the physician is rude or inconsiderate, or worse, that the doctor isn't interested in the patient, doesn't fully understand the nature of the problem, or is incompetent. Similar interpretations may result when a patient is interrupted, or when a physician departs or undertakes various tasks while a patient is speaking.

Also undermining quality communication and relationship development between physicians and patients are missed opportunities to establish rapport. This occurs when customary greetings and closings such as "Hello, how are you today?" or "Goodbye, have a good weekend" are omitted. Impersonal language such as the phrase "How are we feeling?" has now all but become a cliché, and is seen as condescending by many people. Another missed opportunity occurs when a physician fails to use information in a patient's medical record to open an encounter. Consider the following: "Well, I know you were in three months ago for a problem with your arm. How has that been doing?" The message to the patient is likely to be that the physician is thoughtful, interested, informed, and competent.

One of the impactful elements of interpersonal communication is eye contact. The absence of eye contact, common to encounters between physicians and patients, contributes to an impression of disinterest, preoccupation, and depersonalization. On the other hand, the presence of eye contact, even if only at the initial stage and end of an encounter is likely to be read as an indication of interest, attention, and personal concern. Other nonverbal factors either facilitate or impede intended communication outcomes as will be discussed later.

Table 5.6
Questions for Eliciting a Patient's Mental Model
of a Medical Problem

1. What is your problem? How do you describe it?

2. What do you think caused your problem?

3. Why do you think it started when it did?

4. What does your illness do to you?

5. How severe is it?

6. Are the problems short- or long-term?

7. What do you fear most about your problem?

8. What are the major problems your illness has created for you?

9. What kind of treatment do you think you should receive?

10. What are the results you hope for from treatment?

(Source: Arthur Kleinman, *Patients and Healers in the Context of Culture.* (Berkeley: University of California Press, 1980), p. 106.)

Critical Physician Communication Competencies

What, then, are the basic communication competencies that are important for physicians? Perhaps the most basic competence has to do with one's framework for thinking about and approaching encounters with patients. One useful way to think about physician-patient encounters is as in terms of *intercultural* communication. In an intercultural situation, we recognize that we are dealing with individuals with differing backgrounds and often differing language capability. Even where there is a common language – as when we engage in communication with someone from England or Australia – we recognize the limitations of our own slang and colloquialisms. The critical point is that in such situations, we acknowledge that barriers to communication exist and we are careful about the assumptions we make, we ask carefully-selected questions, explain ourselves fully, and in general, exercise considerable effort to be certain that our messages are interpreted as we intend.

This same approach will serve us well in physician-patient encounters, where the intercultural dimensions of the relationship may be easily overlooked simply because it appears the same language is spoken by both parties. Overcoming the barriers in professional-lay encounters often requires considerable "unnatural" effort and "uncommon sense" to break out of the assumptions each party brings to the situation.

Kleinman (1980) suggests that for physicians a fundamental problem in this regard is to gain an understanding of the patient's mental model of his or her medical problem. He suggests a series of questions that may be helpful for bridging cultural barriers. See Table 5.6.

Information-Exchange Competencies

Three other communication competency areas are essential for physicians, the first of which have to do with information exchange. Information exchange competence is necessary to identify patients' clinical _and_ communication needs. Clarity and non-technical language also facilitate accurate and efficient information exchange and retention (Ley, 1983).

Providing opportunities and encouragement for patients to ask questions contributes to accuracy and efficiency of information transfer, as does the use of written as well as oral communication. Finally, sensitivity to nonverbal cues is useful to identify levels of anxiety, understanding, potential confusion, and probability of compliance. See Table 5.7

Compliance-Gaining Competencies

Compliance is enhanced when recommendations are specific, when they are conveyed in both oral and written messages, and when the reasons for a recommendation are fully understood. The more the patient understands the physician's mental model of the medical problem, the more likely he or she is to comply.

Conversely, the more a physician understands the mental model of the patient relative to the problem at hand, the better the physician will be able to negotiate understanding and achieve cooperation in the management of the problem.

Finally, it is often helpful if the physician asks the patient to repeat back his or her understanding of what is being prescribed, and to make commitment to follow through on the recommendation. For instance, a physician might conclude a discussion of recommended medications, life style changes, or follow up procedures by asking the patient what problems he or she sees in following the recommendations? If problems are noted, the physician can address the issues. If not, a commitment can be requested, and the benefits to the patient for compliance can be restated.

Table 5.7
Critical Physician Communication Competencies

- "Intercultural" Thinking

    Different Background
    Different Education
    Different Language
    Different Mental Models
    Different Communication Styles
    Different Perspectives

- Information-Exchange Competencies

    Identify Patient Clinical AND Communication Needs
    Communicate Clearly in Non-Technical Terms
    Encourage Question-Asking
    Use Written and Oral Communication
    Be Sensitive to Nonverbal Cues

- Compliance-Gaining Competencies

    Be Specific
    Explain Reasons for Recommendations
    Repeat and Solicit Paraphrasing
    Ask for Commitment

- Relationship Development and Maintenance Competencies

    Establish Rapport
    Display Interpersonal Sensitivity
    Encourage Openness
    Exhibit Empathy

Relationship Development and Maintenance Competencies

An important objective in any relationship is establishing rapport in order to facilitate information communication and collaboration. As with all relationships, there must be an initiation stage of an encounter during which the physician strives to convey a sense of interest in and concern about the patient.

As an encounter proceeds, the goal is to be sensitive to communication as well as to the clinical aspects of a case in order to anticipate probable reactions, fears, concerns, and to select a communication strategy appropriate to the person and situation. Ideally a climate is created by the physician in which patients feel they can share critical questions, concerns, thoughts, and feelings.

Conveying empathy for the thoughts and feelings of patients is extremely important. Reminding oneself how you would be feeling if this were your father, mother, son, daughter? How would you want them to be treated?

Physician Oliver Sacks (1984, 9. 92), articulately expresses much of this need when he describes his own circumstances when he was a patient:

> What I could not do for myself in a hundred years, precisely because I was entangled in my own patienthood. . . *he* (the physician) could cut across at a single stroke, with the scalpel of detachment, insight and authority. I did not require an actuarial statement, such as "we see this syndrome in 60 per cent of all cases. It has been variously attributed to x, y, and z. The recovery rate is variously estimated as such-and-such, depending on this-and-that, and other imponderables." I required only the voice, the simplicity, the conviction, of authority: "Yes, I understand. It happens. Don't fret. Do this! Believe me! You will soon be well."

> If he could not, in truth, reassure me . . . I would want an honest acknowledgment of the fact. I would equally respect his integrity and authority if he said: "Sacks, it's the damndest thing – I don't know what you've got. But we'll do our best to find out". . . I should respect whatever he said so long as it was frank and showed respect for me, for my dignity as a man.

A number of basic communication skills and sensitivities are important for relationship development and maintenance, information transfer, and compliance gaining. Among these are interpersonal communication style, nonverbal communication sensitivity, patient-centered listening and observation, and confrontation and complaint handling. Each of these will be discussed in the Chapters which follow.

55

Chapter 6

COMMUNICATION STYLE

We take our ability to converse with others very much for granted, so much so that it may seem like quite a simple activity. Clearly, this is not the case. In this and the final three chapters, we will briefly discuss interpersonal concepts, competencies, and strategies that are especially important to caregiver-patient communication. Specifically, our focus will be on:

• Communication Style

• Nonverbal Communication

• Listening, Observation, and Interpretation

• Confrontation, Criticism, and Complaints

Two Contrasting Styles

One way to explore the topic of communication style and its importance for health communication is to distinguish between two quite different communication styles – the "machine-gun" and the "marshmallow."

The "Machine-Gun" Style

The machine-gun style is associated with people whose general approach to dealing with interpersonal situations involves active message sending, as illustrated in Figure 6.1. The style is highly verbal; people who exemplify this style talk a lot and generally say "what's on their minds." There is seldom a need to guess what the machine-gun is thinking or feeling; when a person with this style is upset, happy, angry, or remorseful, you know it.

Figure 6.1

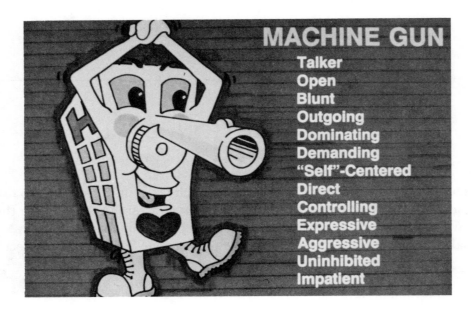

Machine-guns are very expressive. They are generally spontaneous and uninhibited in social situations, and they have little reluctance to voice their opinions, attitudes, or beliefs on topics at hand. Because of their highly expressive and forceful style, they can be controlling, demanding, and dominating.

During a conversation, a machine-gun's attention is focused on what he or she is thinking, how he or she feels, how he or she evaluates the other person's messages, and what he or she wants to say next. As a result, little time or effort is spent focusing on the other person, or in analyzing how his or her own messages are affecting others.

To see how communication style affects health communication, consider the following example:

> One evening Bill is experiencing chest pains and goes to a health center to be seen on an emergency basis. After explaining his situation to the receptionist and filling out the necessary paperwork, he takes a seat in the waiting room, and waits to be called. Twenty minutes pass and he has not yet been seen. However, while he's been waiting two other people have already come and gone.

What does Bill do or say at this point? Bill's behavior will depend largely on his communication style. To the extent that he uses a machine-gun style, he may well approach the desk to point out that he has chest pains, that he has been waiting to be seen for twenty minutes, and that he has noticed that others who have arrived later than he have been seen first. After all, Bill reasons that he is in pain, that this situation could be serious, and

58

Figure 6.2

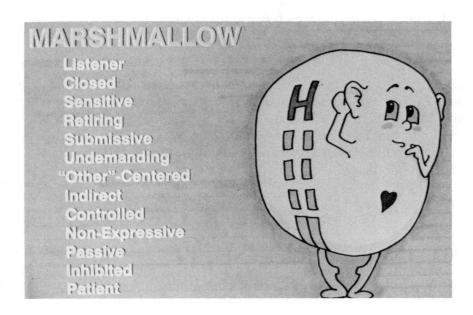

that there's no reason why he shouldn't have been seen by now. If Bill is extreme in his style, he may handle the situation aggressively, either demanding an explanation or insisting on being seen immediately.

The "Marshmallow" Style

In marked contrast are individuals who exemplify what can be termed a marshmallow style, as shown in Figure 6.2 People with this style approach interpersonal situations in a far more passive and restrained manner than machine-guns. They are listeners, and are often "absorbers" of the messages of machine-guns. Unlike machine-guns, one must often guess about the marshmallow's thoughts, opinions, feelings, attitudes, and beliefs. Generally, marshmallow-style communicators are submissive, and often dominated in conversations.

"Marshmallows" are often very cautious about what they say and when and how they say it because they are typically very concerned about how their messages will affect others. They spend a good deal of time planning and analyzing the impact of their message-sending. Accordingly, the marshmallow may be appreciated by others to the extreme of being taken for granted and taken advantage of.

The marshmallow may dislike or even resent this pattern, though he or she is unlikely to express this sentiment openly. Sometimes a build-up of frustration leads the person eventually to "blow-up," often in a manner or circumstance that is confusing to others who may regard the behavior as "out of character."

Think again about the situation in which Bill comes to a health facility for emergency care and waits to be seen while others are taken before him. Assume now that Bill has a marsh-mallow style." How does he react? What does he say?

Quite probably, Bill will not do or say anything at this point but instead will sit patiently "waiting his turn." He might reason that other people may have had problems more serious than his own. Moreover, the staff seems very busy, and he doesn't want to add to their stress. They'll call him as soon as they can. If he were to approach the desk at all, it would be simply to remind the staff in an apologetic tone that he is waiting to be seen in case he had been overlooked.

Caregiver Communication Styles

Up to this point, the examples chosen have focused on *patients'* communication styles and their impact. Obviously, caregivers also have their own communication styles, and these are at least as important to caregiver-patient communication outcomes as the styles of patients.

Consider the following questions:

- What is the most desirable communication style for caregivers?

- What are the strengths and liabilities of the machine-gun style for?

- What are the strengths and liabilities of the marshmallow style?

- What types of patients are easiest for the machine-gun to deal with?

- What types of patients are easiest for the marshmallow to deal with?

- In dealing with machine-gun patients, what are the risks for staff who are machine-guns?

- In dealing with marshmallow patients, what are the risks for staff who are marsh-mallows?

Assets and Liabilities

Both styles have assets and liabilities. As portrayed in Figure 6.3, machine-guns are articulate, direct, open, outgoing, and able to take charge and to provide leadership, and these are certainly attributes that most people admire. Unfortunately, there are also liabilities associated with the machine-gun style, including being potentially too quick to respond, verbally abusive, insensitive, manipulative, and unaware of nonverbal cues.

60

Figure 6.3
"Machine-Gun" Style Assets and Liabilities

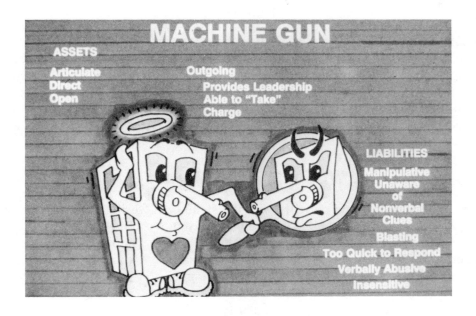

Figure 6.4
"Marshmallow" Style Assets and Liabilities

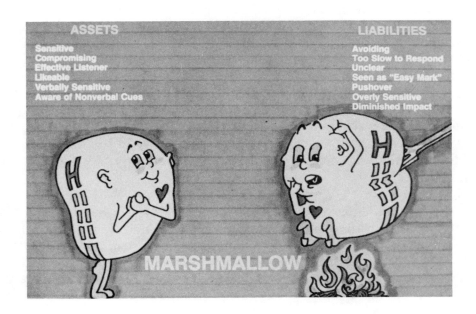

In their training, health caregivers – especially physicians – are generally encouraged to utilize the machine-gun style, rather than the marshmallow style. However, the attributes of the marshmallow style are certainly very much needed and respected in a wide range of health care settings.

Assets of the marshmallow style include being verbally sensitive, being able to compromise, being effective in listening and information gathering, and being likeable and sought out for conversation, as shown in Figure 6.4. However, as with the machine-gun, there are also a number of liabilities associated with the marshmallow style, which include being potentially slow to respond, being unclear and having a diminished impact, being seen as "easy mark" or a pushover, and being overly sensitive.

When Styles Interact

What happens when staff and patients with the same or differing communication styles come into contact with one another? Generally speaking we tend to be most comfortable dealing with persons with styles different from our own. The machine-gun enjoys the passive, supportive listening provided by the marshmallow. And the marshmallow often enjoys the verbal leadership provided by the machine-gun.

In contrast, machine-guns often have difficulty dealing with other machine-guns. Two individuals with this style may collide because both wish to talk and provide leadership. With two marshmallows, the opposite situation may occur, with neither person comfortable being assertive, controlling, or directive.

Often a problem arises, for instance, when a caregiver who usually uses a machine-gun style comes in contact with a machine-gun patient. In the example earlier, for instance, if Bill uses a machine-gun style when he approaches a staff member who is also a machine-gun, sparks – and perhaps a war – may ensure. In such a situation, the caregiver's first impulse is to defend or counterattack, letting Bill know that there are a number of good reasons why he hasn't been seen yet, and that he should sit and wait his turn patiently. This may well accentuate Bill's machine-gunning, which in turn may trigger more machine-gunning by the caregiver. The eventual result, of course, is dissatisfaction for Bill *and* for the caregiver, as well as the potential for a negative impact on reputations, the lodging of formal follow-up complaints, and most importantly, the potential for compromised health care.

A situation such as this underscores the need for caregivers to be aware of their own communication style, sensitive to its assets and liabilities, and flexible enough to make adjustments in that style when a situation warrants it. For instance, the best strategy for dealing with a machine-gun as in the situation above is to adopt a more marshmallow style, to diffuse the machine-gun and to create an atmosphere where reasoned conversation is possible, as shown in Figure 6.5.

Figure 6.5

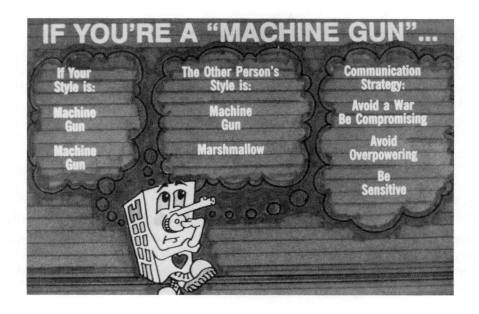

Figure 6.6

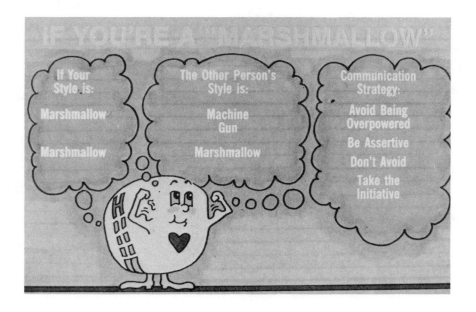

Difficulties can also arise for machine-guns dealing with marshmallows in a caregiver-patient situation. This is especially so if a machine-gun assumes that others are not in need of particular attention because they are passive and undemanding. In this kind of situation, the machine-gun is likely to assume that if others around them have serious problems, they'll let those problems be known, but particularly with individuals who use a marshmallow style, this will often not be the case. To return again to the example of Bill, imagine this time that the caregiver is a machine-gun, but Bill is a marshmallow. Bill may well sit patiently with worsening chest pains, rather than returning to the desk to advise caregivers of his worsening condition.

With caregivers who tend most often to use a marshmallow style, the greatest difficulty comes in dealing with machine-gun patients, who can easily be overwhelming inter-personally. The tendency in such instances is to avoid being overpowered and to push oneself to be assertive. See Figure 6.6.

Neither style is appropriate in all circumstances. In some situations, and with some people, the machine-gun style is probably most advantageous. In other circumstances, and with other people, the marshmallow is more appropriate. Often, the best strategy is a blend of the two. The ideal, therefore, is to be be aware and flexible enough to use the machine-gun style, the marshmallow style, or a combination, depending upon the circumstance.

Specifically, caregivers can benefit from:

- Knowing their usual and/or preferred communication style.

- Knowing the kinds of patients, colleagues, and situations for which their ususal style works well, and those for which it does not.

- Striving to broaden their "communication style comfort zone" in order to have a range of options available.

- Selecting a communication style based on its appropriateness to the people and to the situation, rather than one based on habit.

Chapter 7

NONVERBAL COMMUNICATION

Nonverbal messages are often even more important than verbal messages to interpersonal relations. Nonverbal messages arise from people's appearance, facial expressions, eye behavior, dress, gestures, touch, and tone of voice. These messages play the central role in caregiver-patient communication. Particularly in the formation of first impressions, or where there are conflicts between someone's words and actions, nonverbal communication is often far more influential than verbal communication.

Typically, verbal messages are used to send various kinds of content messages – generally information – that a sender purposely chooses to send. Nonverbal messages, such as looking away while speaking to someone, a frown, or a rushed or brusque tone, are often created unintentionally. Even though nonverbal messages may be sent accidentally they can be very important. Whether intended or not, looking away while someone is speaking is likely to be interpreted as disinterest, a frown as disapproval, and a brusque tone as annoyance.

Researcher Albert Mehrabian (1971, pp. 42-47) indicates that where we are uncertain about how we feel about another person, verbal messages account for only seven percent of our overall impression, the remainder being accounted for by nonverbal factors:

Total Impression = 7% Verbal Messages + 38% Vocal Messages + 55% Facial Messages

Differences Between Verbal and Nonverbal Codes

Compared to verbal communication, there is a general lack of awareness of the nonverbal communication. Only during the last several decades has there been a recognition of the important role nonverbal communication plays. Even today, there is a dramatic contrast between the relative attention given to verbal, as compared to nonverbal, communication in the educational process. Verbal communication proficiency is considered to be one of the basic skills, and taught in one form or another in every grade; nonverbal skills receive little or no attention in most schools.

One of the explanations for the emphasis placed on verbal communication is that the rules for using oral and written language are very explicit compared to nonverbal communication. Information about language structure and usage is available in any number of sources, from style manuals to dictionaries. However, nothing comparable exists for nonverbal communication.

Nonetheless, there are any number of agreed upon rules for nonverbal communication which we learn indirectly through observation. There are rules about what to to do and not do in particular situations, what to wear, how to greets others, how close to stand to others while conversing, when touch is appropriate in interpersonal relations, and what various tones of voice convey. However, few of us give much conscious thought to these rules that guide our interpersonal behavior in social settings.

For health caregivers, some conscious attention to the nonverbal communication, the rules which guide our nonverbal behavior, and the potential uses of nonverbal messages can be very valuable. For caregivers, nonverbal communication is a valuable supplement to verbal communication for identifying and confirming patients' feelings, thoughts, concerns, and fears. For patients, who come to a health care situation with anxiety, uncertainty, and confusion nonverbal messages are often the primary basis for making sense of a caregiver and of the situation.

Types of Nonverbal Communication

In the sections ahead, we will briefly consider the following types of nonverbal communication: appearance, facial expressions, eye behavior, dress, gestures, touch, and tone of voice.

Appearance

It is said that "Beauty is only skin-deep," and "You can't judge a book by its cover." However, there is little doubt that when other sources of information are lacking, "surface-level" messages play a critical role in human communication. Particularly in the formation of initial impressions, appearance is probably the single most important factor. A number of factors contribute to our judgments of appearance, among them face, hair, eyes, physique, dress, and adornment.

Generally speaking, we react to a person's face and facial expressions as a whole. Researchers believe that the role of the face in relation to the expression of emotion is common to all humans. Paul Ekman (1972, p. 216) explains: "What is universal in facial expressions of emotion is the particular set of facial muscular movements when a given emotion is elicited." The specific circumstances that lead to the expression of emotions vary from one individual and one culture to another. The emotions evoked by ceremonies accompanying death, for instance, may vary greatly from one person to another depending upon the individual's personality and the way the event is viewed in the given culture.

Based on a person's face – often influenced greatly by the presence or absence of a smile – we make fairly global assessments of the individual, his or her attitudes and emotions relative to us, and his or her feelings relative to a situation at hand. For most of us, a smile is a very powerful "signal," one that creates an expectation of a satisfying encounter and an atmosphere of receptivity to verbal communication.

The elements of the face which generally have the most impact in terms of nonverbal communication are the eyes. When conversing with even a casual acquaintance, some degree of mutual eye contact is expected. Indeed, this is one of the unwritten rules of interpersonal communication competence. In such circumstances, "looking" may help grasping the ideas being discussed. Eye contact is often taken as an indication of attention and interest by receivers, a particularly important goal in caregiver-patient interaction. In these and other situations, the absence of contact reduces the likelihood of interaction. Eye gaze also plays an important role in personal attraction. Generally speaking, positive feelings toward an individual and high degree of eye contact go together. Perhaps for this reason, we generally assume that people who look our way are attracted to us. Individuals who engage in high levels of eye contact are typically also seen as interpersonally influential and effective.

Dress fulfills a number of purposes for us, including decoration, physical and psychological protection, attraction, self-assertion, group identification, and display of status or role. Cosmetics, jewelry, eyeglasses, and hair styles serve many of these same goals. Because of their many functions, dress and adornment are often used as the basis for interpersonal impressions.

Note the number of impressions that might be drawn from the nonverbal messages in the photos in Figure 7.1. Consider the range of reactions caregivers might have to each of these individuals were they to appear as patients at a hospital, HMO, clinic, or group practice. In everyday communication situations, dress and jewelry is an important means of self expression. Dress follows individual, group, occupational, and cultural rules. These rules guide us in our choices of dress and they guide others in the interpretations they make of us for better or worse.

It is important to recognize that many of the normal rules of everyday nonverbal communication are violated in health care settings, and perhaps none so dramatically as dress. Caregivers may be accustomed to these "rule violations" while patients are not. Dress is used to send a variety of messages – about one's wealth, occupation, and identity. Dress may be a way of saying: "This is who I am"; "Notice me"; "I'm important"; or "Pay attention to me." In a health care setting, often this form of self-expression is often severely limited. For many patients the necessity of undressing and having to encounter caregivers dressed in hospital gowns is quite distressing, since a familiar way of expressing one's identity to others is quite literally stripped away. Not surprisingly, the result can be considerable discomfort, disorientation, and a sense of loss of control. Thus, to the extent possible, it is desirable to begin caregiver-patient encounters when a patient is dressed.

Figure 6.1

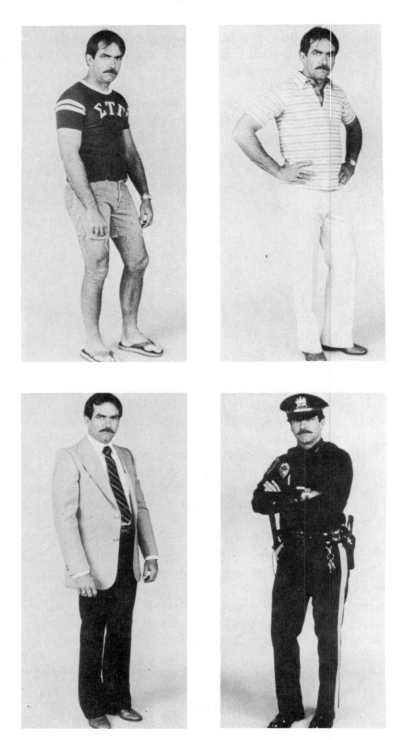

Chapter 8

Listening, Observing, and Interpreting

Observation, interpretation and listening are often at least as important in caregiver-patient communication as are communication style and nonverbal communication. Competence in these areas is needed in order to get the information that is necessary to provide appropriate medical care: At the same time, listening, observation, and interpretation are ways of conveying a sense of interest and concern for the patient.

Selection, Interpretation, Retention

Listening, observing, and interpreting are basic and familiar aspects of human communication. As simple and automatic as these may seem, each involves a complex of factors operating in a very active process of message selection, message interpretation, and message retention (Ruben, 1992b).

Message Selection

At any instant in time, we are surrounded by a number of persons, objects, and circumstances which are the sources of the messages that compete for our attention and interest. From these potential sources, we select certain cues to listen to and observe while disregarding others. The simplicity of the activity often obscures its complexity.

To say we select may be somewhat misleading because it implies that this is something we do purposefully, when most often it is a natural process of which we are largely unaware. Message selection operates in all kinds of common situations, such as when we pause in a hallway to chat with a colleague. The very act of noticing the other person involves the systematic selection of a message. Triggered by a number of factors associated with the appearance of the other person, and perhaps a verbal message – "Hi!" – we begin tuning ourselves in to the other person and to the messages necessary to the encounter which will follow. In so doing, we ignore other potential messages – the temperature, the color of the carpeting, the appearance of other persons who may pass by, the noise of a nearby copy machine, or the thunderstorm outside.

In some situations the selective nature of observation and listening is apparent, as when we read a book or talk with friends in a room with a stereo or television set turned on or a lawn mower running outside. In these circumstances, we selectively listen to or observe certain messages while disregarding others,that we define as background noise. Another illustration of the selective nature of message reception is provided by cocktail parties and similar social gatherings. During such affairs, one finds that it is not at all difficult to carry on a series of perfectly intelligible discussions with one or more individuals without being overly distracted by other conversations. It is even possible to tune in to an exchange between several other individuals a good distance away without shifting one's position and while appearing to be deeply engrossed in conversation with a person close at hand. In that same setting, we are able to tune out the entire external environment, periodically, in order to concentrate on our own feelings, decide what we ought to be doing, or think about how we are being perceived by others.

In most other situations, however, selection is not a process we think much about, and herein lies a number of potential risks. To the extent that we are guided mostly by our habits and previous experiences in our decisions about what to listen to or to observe, it is quite possible that we will miss potentially valuable sources of information.

Interpretation

A second facet of reception is the interpretation of messages. When we interpret messages we determine what significance to attach to a word, sentence, circumstance, gesture, or event, and how to respond – whether to regard it as fiction or nonfiction, serious or humorous, new or old, contradictory or consistent, amusing or annoying. Even our reaction to a simple statement such as, "Hi, how are you?" will depend on a number of factors and the meanings we attach to them: whether, for instance, the person is male or female (and the significance we attach to each), whether we regard the individual as attractive or unattractive, whether he or she is a patient or a physician, whether we are at a hospital or a sporting event, whether the person is dressed in swimwear or uniform, whether we are situated on nearby blankets at the beach or next to one another in a doctor's waiting room, whether we interpret the individual's motives as platonic or clinical, and a number of other factors.

For the most part, our interpretations of particular events, objects, words, appearances, dress, and gestures are dictated by the message reception rules and habits we have learned over time.

Retention – Memory

Memory plays an indispensable role in the interpretative process. We are able to store and actively use an incredible amount of information – at least several billion times more than a large research computer – and yet we can locate and use it with an efficiency and ease of operation that is astounding. We have little difficulty accessing the information we need in order to go about our daily routine – to remember our address, phone number, and how to get to our place of work, how to start and operate an automobile, and how to perform the many duties required in our positions.

Some Factors That Influence Listening, Observation, and Interpretation

For each of us a complex set of elements work together to influence our decisions as to which kinds of messages we hear and observe and how we will interpret and retain the meanings that result. While some external factors come into play, many of these influences have to do with the nature of the individual receiver.

For instance, the preferences, attitudes, opinions, predispositions, and habits one has regarding particular topics, persons, or situations play a critical role in observing and listening and in the interpretations that result. The tendency in message reception is to attend to and be favorably disposed toward messages, messages sources, and interpretations which support their existing views and our experience before considering alternative messages, sources, or conclusions.

In a similar manner, our goals – to become a physician or nurse, for instance – direct our attention toward certain sorts of messages and away from others. The aspiring doctor or nurse is directed by his or her goal toward a knowledge base in physiology, anatomy, chemistry and away from messages that would be more pertinent to students of engineering, business administration, and journalism. Acquiring appropriate interpretations for these messages is crucial, and it is a priority until the goal is met or changed. Interestingly enough, even a change of goals often involves observation, listening, and interpretation.

Another factor which influences listening, observation, and interpretation is *use.* Generally speaking, people are likely to observe, listen to, and devote effort to understand and remember messages that they think they will need or be able to use. Therefore, in assessing a patient's condition, a physician pays particular attention to those messages he or she has learned through training and experience will be useful information in making a diagnosis.

Habit and experience are also major guiding forces in listening, observation, and interpretation. In each of these examples mentioned above, one can see the extent to which characteristics of the receiver are important in message reception – and for good and understandable reasons. Often, however, receiver-centered factors become so influential that they can overshadow or even obscure other factors that should be equally important considerations – the sender's perspective, for instance. By implication, one can see how

Figure 8.1
Observation and Interpretation:
A Matter of Point of View and Perspective

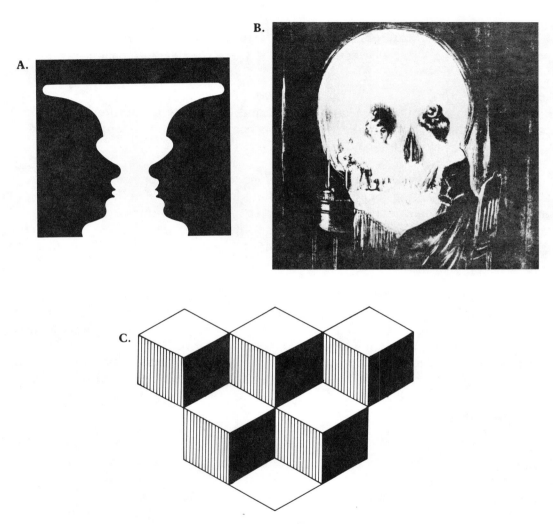

Figure 8.1 provides graphic illustrations of the well-worn but still significant adage, "there is always more than one way to look at things." In health care as in other contexts, one's needs, uses, point of view, experience, and other attributes shape what we see and the interpretations that result. In Figure 8.1 are we seeing a vase or two faces staring at one another, an X-ray of a skull or a woman seated at a dressing table looking at herself in the mirror, five cubes or three cubes? Not surprisingly, caregivers and patients often look at and interpret their "common" health care experiences in very different ways.

the needs, opinions, goals, and anticipated information uses of a caregiver can lead to caregiver-centered listening and observation which unintentionally tunes out patients' needs, attitudes, goals, and anticipated information uses. To the extent that this occurs, the communication process and the encounter may be effective for the caregiver, but it is likely not to be nearly as satisfying or productive from the receiver's perspective.

"Caregiver-Centered" vs. "Patient-Centered" Listening

For the reasons discussed above, "patient-centered" listening is often a challenge, requiring sensitivity to the needs and perspectives of the patient first and foremost. Without making a concerted effort to be patient-centered, the more natural dynamics of listening occur resulting in the following patterns:

• Listening inattentively unless the content is of special importance to the listener.

• Asking few questions unless they are essential to the needs and goals of the listener .

• Assuming a knowledge of what a sender is going to say before he or she has finished speaking.

• Jumping quickly to agree or disagree with what is being said.

• Thinking about what he or she is going to say next while the other person is talking.

• Interrupting.

• Looking around while being spoken to.

• "Listening" while thinking about or doing other things.

This form of "listening" is generally not effective for either for gathering accurate information or for creating a positive interpersonal climate. By way of contrast, "patient centered" listening involves:

• Listening actively, recognizing that effective listening is difficult.

• Looking like you're listening – eye contact and body position – to enhance the clarity of verbal and nonverbal interpretations

• Asking open-ended questions rather than questions which can simply be answered with a "yes" or "no."

• Restating and paraphrasing what you think you heard to confirm listening accuracy, to heighten the probably mutual understanding, and to exude a sense of empathy.

• Avoiding hasty responses and delay personal judgments or evaluations of the "adequacy" or "inadequacy," "appropriateness" or "inappropriateness" of what the other person is saying.

Chapter 9

Confrontation, Criticism, and Complaints

The need to respond appropriately and effectively to patient and family complaints is increasingly critical in health care organizations of all kinds. A number of factors give urgency to this need.

• Effective January 1, 1990 health care facilities accredited by the Joint Commission on Accreditation of Healthcare Organizations (JCAHO) will be required to have formalized procedures in place for dealing with patient complaints. Specifically, the standards require procedures for receiving complaints, informing patients of their right to file a complaint, responding to significant complaints with appropriate actions, and assuring that patients who complain will not suffer negative consequences.

• Today's health care consumers are better educated and certainly more demanding than in previous periods. Complaints have become a common form of self-expression and assertiveness, an increasingly acceptable way of registering dissatisfaction, even a way of attempting to demonstrate one's knowledge or expertise.

• Concerns regarding the quality of healthcare, healthcare personnel, and healthcare system, in general are on the public agenda. A recent Louis Harris Poll, for instance, finds that 8 of 9 citizens believe the U. S. health-care system needs a major overhaul (USA Today, May 25, 1989).

• Increasing competition among providers underscores the values of patient satisfaction and the costs of dissatisfaction.

• A complaint is often an early warning sign of potential litigation to follow. The way complaints are handled may well have an impact on the likelihood of subsequent litigation.

Criticism and Complaints as Opportunities

Improved understanding and skill in interpersonal and written communication is vital in order to be able to respond appropriately and effectively to confrontation, complaints, and criticism, and more generally, to increase patient and family satisfaction, confidence, and trust.

Caregivers must come to regard these situations as a challenge rather than simply a problem. Confrontations, criticism, and complaints are an opportunity to learn about patient perceptions, patient evaluative criteria, potential health care policy or procedural problems, and an opportunity to transform a dissatisfied consumer. Research evidence shows that when complaints from dissatisfied consumers are handled well, those individuals become more vocal, positive, and loyal consumers than other customers who have been satisfied all along.

In the case of patients, confrontations, criticism, and complaints may result from frustration, anger, confusion, or annoyance, and generally a combination of all three. Very often, a patient's feelings are not directed at the person toward whom the hostility, criticism, or complaint is addressed. Sometimes the recipient just happens to be the nearest person at a time of particular frustration or anxiety for a patient. Nonetheless, caregivers are confronted with expressions of hostility and criticism, and the understandable tendency is to react negatively and generally to take criticism and complaints personally.

The tendency is to *defend* – especially when we are prone to a machine-gun communication style – or to *withdraw* or *avoid* – particularly if the marshmallow style is customary for us. Unless he or she has an understanding of interpersonal communication and self-awareness, the caregiver with a machine-gun style is likely to react to a patient complaint or criticism with an immediate verbal defense or a counter-attack. Since machine-gun patients are more likely to complain than marshmallows, the confrontation is likely to lead to "a war." Frequently, the result is that the patient is not only annoyed about the initial problem, but also about the way his or her complaint was handled. Hostility builds and the problem intensifies. The marshmallow, on the other hand, might feel overpowered in such a situation and cope by "avoiding," withdrawing and saying little or nothing. Neither extreme works well.

What often works very well as a way of responding to confrontations, criticism, and complaints is the communication strategy outlined in Figure 9.1. This approach is generally quite effective because it 1) helps to clarify the exact nature of the problem being addressed, and 2) because the overriding message conveyed by the caregiver is one of concern for the patient. Since a perceived lack of concern is usually one of the factor motivating confrontation, criticism, or complaint in the first place, an expression of concern does much to shift the encounter to a more positive and productive plane.

Figure 9.1
Communication Strategies for Responding To Confrontations, Criticism, and Complaints

---

1. Acknowledge understanding of specific complaints by restating key points.

2. Acknowledge legitimacy of feelings.

3. Address concerns, provide information, and/or specify actions or steps.

4. Clarify intentions and goals.

5. Apologize for the problem or inconvenience.

6. Thank individual for taking the time and effort to share his or her concern.

7. Encourage future comment and suggestions.

Face-to-Face Confrontation

Consider how the steps in this approach would be applied in the following face-to-face situations, and how successful a caregiver using the strategy might be in fostering a more positive, productive, and mutually satisfying climate for discussion.

• Patient: "I've been ignored for 45 minutes while you've taken care of other patients who came after me. I've had it. Who's in charge here? I want to talk to him."

• Patient: "I called thirty minutes ago. I was promised that Dr. Smith would call me back immediately. Why haven't I heard from him? I can't stay here waiting for the telephone call. I'm a very busy person. Can't you understand that? There's simply no excuse for your incompetence!"

• After weeks of pain and visits to several physicians, a patient has been referred to a "highly-regarded specialist." The patient introduces herself and begins to describe her symptoms. The physician explains that it isn't necessary to hear her symptoms, that the examination and test results will tell him everything he will need to know. An irate husband calls to complain: "When my wife goes to a specialist after waiting many weeks to get in and paying the price you charge, I don't expect her to be treated abruptly and made to feel like an idiot."

• A patient diagnosed as having an extensive tear in his lateral meniscus is told by one orthopedic surgeon that he should be back to work within a week to ten days at most. A second physician tells him it may be 4 to 6 weeks before he'll be back to work. The patient becomes angry. "What? The other doctor said it would be a week. What the hell is going on here?"

81

Written Complaints

Confrontation, criticism, and complaints also occur in written communication between caregivers and patients, as exemplified by the complaint letter provided in Figure 9.2. How should one respond to a letter such as this kind of criticism? One typical response is provided in Figure 9.3. What weaknesses are present in this response? Some limitations are listed in Figure 9.4.

What kind of letter would result from applying the communication strategy discussed in Figure 9.1? Figure 9.5 provides a version of a response letter based on this framework, and Figure 9.6 presents the same letter with superscripts to indicate which steps in the strategy outlined in Figure 9.1 particular sentences and phrases exemplify.

Figure 9.2
Complaint Letter

JANE JOHNSON
14 DISSATISFACTION DRIVE
PRINCETON, NEW JERSEY

August 31, 1992

Dr. Bird, M.D.
Health Center
Ocean City, NJ 08502

Dear Dr. Bird:

What do you have to do to get standard health care with dignity for patients at your health center?? I'm talking about <u>appointments</u> for certain levels of injury and care under <u>all circumstances,</u> including during the summer.

I suffered a head injury on an airline which almost required stitches and was bleeding for several hours. I thought once I got back to the States, I could receive some attention for my injury in the form of a scheduled appointment, required shots ,and follow-up appointment. Pretty basic, huh? I thought so. But your operation insisted on making me fight to get a set time to see a physician. Moreover, after recommending a tetanus shot they didn't have the vaccine stored and the pharmacy was closed at the time.

So it was recommended I return in 5 days. This left me unprotected for sometime, yet when I suggested setting up a time for the visit, again I was rebuffed. What's with you people? I'm between a rock and a hard place because this is my <u>only</u> health plan and I can't afford to go elsewhere. So I'm forced to be treated like cattle no matter how severe my injury, instead of getting the dignity of a scheduled appointment for my care and treatment.

This, I think you would agree, is a ridiculous and ludicrous policy and deserves to be reconsidered by you and your staff. Certain levels of health care – including head injuries – deserve certain levels of treatment including the dignity of an appointment upon request. I look forward to hearing your thoughts on this matter and what you plan to do about my concerns.

Sincerely,

Jane Johnson

cc: President Allen,
   Dr. Waltersberg
   Dr. Servero

Figure 9.3
Response Letter No. 1

Health Service
4 Care Road
Princeton, New Jersey

October 23, 1992

Jane Johnson
14 Dissatisfaction Drive
Princeton, New Jersey

Dear Jane:

I am writing concerning the letter you sent to Dr. Bird on August 31, 1989. A patient representative has already talked with you concerning this matter, but I felt it best if I also wrote to you.

I know that you were upset and concerned because of your head injury. It is my understanding that you received first aid treatment for this injury when it had occurred three days prior to your visit to the health center. Therefore, this was not an emergency, but an urgent visit. The staff still treated you as a priority patient by not making you wait and by thoroughly evaluating you. If you had waited for an appointment, you would have been seen two to three days later. I don't believe you would have wanted to wait that long to be reevaluated for your injury.

After evaluating the situation both by reviewing your chart and discussing it with those clinicians involved, I do believe you were given adequate and thorough care.

Sincerely,

Frederick Wilson, Director

cc: President Allen,
    Dr. Waltersberg
    Dr. Servero

Figure 9.4
Limitations of Response Letter No. 1

1. <u>Impersonal tone</u>.

2. <u>Partially addressed clinical concerns, but not human concerns</u>. The original letter included reference to "health care with dignity" suggesting that this patient's complaint had to do with both clinical and communication issues. Note that this is usually the case with letters of complaint in health care.

3. <u>Lack of empathy displayed</u>. The letter fails to include any acknowledgement of patient's feelings. Moreover, telling the patient her circumstance was "not an emergency" when obviously it was an emergency from the patient's perspective is insensitive if not incorrect. The more correct statement would suggest that it was not an emergency as defined in clinical terms and/or in terms of the health center policies, which is quite a different matter, and one which is probably best left unstated to the patient. Including such a statement in a letter of response is certain to further confirm the patient's sense that the center and its staff "treat people like cattle," and would probably only aggravate the situation.

4. <u>Fails to regard this complaint as an opportunity</u> – The letter of complaint provides an opportunity to learn about patients' perceptions and evaluative criteria, to learn of potential policy or procedural problems, and to appease a dissatisfied consumer. Research evidence shows that when complaints written by dissatisfied consumers are handled well, those individuals become more vocal, positive, and loyal consumers than those who are initially satisfied. This letter of response amounts to a lost opportunity and a further exacerbation of the dissatisfaction level of the patient.

5. <u>Discourages future comment by this patient</u>.

6. <u>Fails to deal constructively with the potentially discrediting impact of the letter among other individuals who were sent copies of the latter</u>. The audience for the response letter is not only the patient, but also all others who read the original letter and who will read the response. The response represents a missed opportunity to maintain and/or strengthen relationships and credibility.

Figure 9.5
An Alternative Response Letter

Health Service
4 Care Road
Princeton, New Jersey

October 23, 1992

Jane Johnson
14 Dissatisfaction Drive
Princeton, New Jersey

Dear Jane:

I am writing concerning the letter you sent to Dr. Bird on August 31, 1989. Jim Jameson, our patient representative, has already talked with you concerning this matter, but I wanted to contact you myself as well.

From your letter and discussions with Jim, I am very aware that you were dissatisfied with care you received at our health center, and I certainly have a sense of the frustration you felt. You noted in your letter that you believe you should be able to expect high quality health care with dignity. I certainly agree with this statement, and we are concerned that you feel it was not provided in this case.

It is my understanding that you called our health center to schedule an appointment for first aid for a head injury you had received on an international flight. Instead of providing a specific appointment time as you requested, a staff member recommended that you come in and wait to be seen when a clinician was available. In checking with the people involved, I learned that our staff suggested this because they were treating you as a high priority patient. They knew that by stopping in and waiting you would have been seen more quickly than if an appointment were scheduled. Obviously, all of our good intentions either weren't well communicated or else didn't meet your expectations. We should have checked to be certain that you understood the reason for our recommendation, and if you still preferred an appointment recognizing it might mean you wouldn't be seen as soon, we certainly could have honored your request.

Your annoyance about the lack of availability of tetanus vaccine is also understandable. As I am sure you can understand, periodically supplies do run out, and the pharmacy does operate on a limited schedule during the summer months. However, be assured that neither of these circumstances would have prevented us from getting you the inoculation immediately, if it had been necessary to your treatment. What may not have been made as clear as it should have been was that receiving the vaccine in five days would not present any health risks to you.

86

I can assure you that our goal at our health center is to provide high quality clinical and personal treatment to each and every one of our patients. In this instance, our system didn't work to your satisfaction, and for that we do apologize. We are continually looking for ways to improve the care we provide, and your comments have helped us identify areas in which we need to work to more fully achieve our goals.

Thank you for taking the time to bring your criticisms to our attention. We hope that your next visit to the health center will be much more pleasant, and that you'll continue to feel free to share with me any suggestions you may have as to how we can better serve your health care needs.

Sincerely,

Frederick Wilson, Director

cc: President Allen,
    Dr. Waltersberg
    Dr. Servero

Figure 9.6
An Alternative Response Letter: Coded Version

```
                    Health Service
                    4 Care Road
              Princeton, New Jersey
```

October 23, 1992

Jane Johnson
14 Dissatisfaction Drive
Princeton, New Jersey

Dear Jane:

I am writing concerning the letter you sent to Dr. Bird on August 31, 1989. Jim Jameson, our patient representative, has already talked with you concerning this matter, but I wanted to contact you myself as well.

From your letter and discussions with Jim, I am very aware that you were dissatisfied with care you received at our health center, and I certainly have a sense of the frustration you felt.[2] You noted in your letter that you believe you should be able to expect high quality health care with dignity.[1] I certainly agree with this statement, and we are concerned that you feel it was not provided in this case.

It is my understanding that you called our health center to schedule an appointment for first aid for a head injury you had received on an international flight. Instead of providing a specific appointment time as your requested, a staff member recommended that you come in and wait to be seen when a clinician was available.[1] In checking with the people involved, I learned that our staff suggested this because they were treating you as a high priority patient.[3] They knew that by stopping in and waiting you would have been seen more quickly than if an appointment were scheduled. Obviously, all of our good intentions either weren't well communicated or else didn't meet your expectations.[3,4] We should have checked to be certain that you understood the reason for our

recommendation, and if you still preferred an appointment recognizing it might mean you wouldn't be seen as soon, we certainly could have honored your request.[3]

88

Your annoyance about the lack of availability of tetanus vaccine is also understandable.[1,2] *As I am sure you can understand, periodically supplies do run out, and the pharmacy does operate on a limited schedule during the summer months.*[3]

However, be assured that neither of these circumstances would have prevented us from getting you the inoculation immediately, if it had been necessary to your treatment.[3] *What must not have been made as clear as it should have been was that receiving the vaccine in five days would not present any health risks to you.*[3]

I can assure you that our goal at our health center is to provide high quality clinical and personal treatment to each and every one of our patients.[4] *In this instance, our system didn't work to your satisfaction, and for that we do apologize.*[5] *We are continually looking for ways to improve the care we provide,*[4] *and your comments have helped us identify areas in which we need to work to more fully achieve our goals.*[3]

Thank you for taking the time to bring your criticisms to our attention.[6] *We hope that your next visit to the health center will be much more pleasant, and that you'll continue to feel free to share with me any suggestions you may have as to how we can better serve your health care needs.*[7]

Sincerely,

Frederick Wilson, Director

cc: President Allen,
    Dr. Waltersberg
    Dr. Servero

References and Suggested Readings

Albrecht, T. L. & Adelman, M. B. (1987). *Communication social support.* Newbury Park, CA: Sage.

Argyle, M. (1983). Doctor-patient skills. In D. Pendleton & J. Hasler (Eds.), *Doctor-patient communication* (pp. 57-74). New York: Academic Press.

Ben-Sira, Z. (1990). Primary care practitioners' likelihood to engage in a bio-psychosocial approach: An additional perspective on the doctor-patient relationship. *Social Science and Medicine,* 31(5), 565-576.

Bertakis, K. D. (1977). The communication of information from physician to patient: A method for increasing patient retention and satisfaction. *Journal of Family Practice,* 5(2), 217-222.

Bostrom, R. N. (1984). *Competence in communication.* Newbury Park, CA: Sage.

Burgoon, J. K., & Saine, T. (1978). *The unspoken dialogue.* Boston: Houghton Mifflin.

Bowman, J. C., & Ruben, B. D. (1986). Patient satisfaction: Critical issues in the implementation and evaluation of patient relations training. *Journal of health care Education and Training,* 1(2), 24-27.

Brown, S. W., & Morley, A. P., Jr. (1988). *Marketing strategies for physicians.* Oradell, NJ: Medical Economics Books.

Cline, R. J. (1983). Interpersonal communication skills for enhancing physician-patient relationships. *Maryland State Medical Journal,* April, 272-278.

Cockerham, W. C. (1989). *Medical sociology.* 4th. ed. Englewood Cliffs, NJ: Prentice Hall.

DiMatteo, M. R., & DiNicola, D. D. (1982). *Achieving patient compliance: The psychology of the medical practitioner's role.* New York: Pergamon.

Droste, T. (1988). Quality care: Elusive concept deserves defining. *Hospitals,* April 15, 58-59.

Ekman, P., Friesen, W. V., & Ellsworth, P. (1972). *Human face: Guidelines for research and an integration of the findings.* New York: Pergamon Press.

Ellmer, R., & Olbrisch, M. E. (1983). The contribution of a cultural perspective in understanding and evaluating client satisfaction. *Evaluation and Program Planning,* 6, 275-281.

Engel, G. L. (1979). The biopsychosocial model and the education of health professionals. *General Hospital Psychiatry,* 156-165.

Ernstene, A. C. (1957). Explaining to the patient: A therapeutic tool and professional obligation. *Journal of the American Medical Association,* (November 2), 1110-1113.

Fine, V. F., & Therrien, M. E. (1977). Empathy in the doctor-patient relationship: Skill training for medical studies. *Journal of Medical Education,* 52(752).

Frankel, R., & Beckman, H. (1989). Evaluating the patient's primary problem(s). In M. Stewart & D. Roter (Eds.), *Communication with medical patients* (pp. 86-98). Newbury Park, CA: Sage.

Friedman, E., Katcher, A. H., Lynch, J. J., & Thomas, S. A. (1980). Animal companions and one-year survival of patients after discharge from a coronary care unit. *Public Health Reports,* 95, 307-312.

Garrity, T. F., Stallones, L., Marx, M. B., & Johnson, T. P. (1989). Pet ownership and attachment as supportive factors in the health of the elderly. *Anthrozoos,* 3, 35-44.

Gilman, S. L. (1988). *Disease and representation: Images of illness from madness to AIDS.* Ithaca, NY: Cornell University Press.

Gibbs, N. (1989). Sick and tired: Uneasy patients may Be surprised to find their doctors are worried too. *Time,* July 31, 48-53

Goffman, E. (1971). *Relations in public.* New York: Harper.

Greenfield, S., Kaplan, S., & Ware, J. E. (1985). Expanding patient involvement in care: Effects on patient outcomes. *Annals of Internal Medicine,* 102, 520-528.

Greenfield, S., Kaplan, S., & Ware, J. E. (1986). Expanding patient involvement in care: Effects on Blood Sugar. *Annals of Internal Medicine,* 34(2), 819A.

Gudykunst, W. B. (1991). *Bridging differences.* Newbury Park, CA: Sage.

Haug, M., & Lavin, B. (1983). *Consumerism in medicine: Challenging physician authority.* Beverly Hills, CA: Sage.

Health Communication. A quarterly journal published by Lawrence Erlbaum Associates. Hillsdale, NJ.

Healthy America: Practitioners for 2005 (1991). A report of the Pew Health Professions Commission. Durham, NC: Duke University Medical Center.

Herrling, J. L. (1986). *Student adaptation to a community college.* Rutgers University, New Brunswick, NJ: Graduate School of Education doctoral dissertation.

Hulka, B. S., Kupper, L. L., Cassel, J. C., & Mayo, F. (1975). Doctor-patient communication and outcomes among diabetic patients. *Journal of Community Health,* 1(1), 15-27.

Inui, T. S., Yourtee, E. L., & Williamson, J. W. (1976). Improved outcomes in hypertension after physician tutorials. *Annals of Internal Medicine,* 84, 646-651.

Kaplan, S. H., Greenfield, S., & Ware, J. E. (1989). Assessing the effects of physician-patient interactions on the outcomes of chronic disease. *Medical Care,* 27(3), (Supplement), S110-S127.

Kelly, E. W. J. (1979). *Effective interpersonal communication: A manual for skill development.* Washington, DC: University Press of America.

Kleinman, A. (1980). *Patients and healers in the context of culture: An exploration of the borderland between anthropology, medicine, and psychiatry.* Berkeley, CA: University of California Press.

Knapp, M. L., & Hall, J. A. (1992). *Nonverbal communication in human interaction.* 3rd. ed. Fort Worth, TX: Holt Rinehart & Winston.

Knapp, M. L., & Vangelista, A. L. (1992). *Interpersonal communication and human relations.* 2d. ed. Boston: Allyn and Bacon.

Klinzing, D., & Klinzing, D. (1985). *Communication for allied health professionals.* Dubuque, IA: Wm. C. Brown.

Korsch, B. M., & Gozzi, E. K. (1968). Gaps in doctor-patient communication: I. Doctor-patient interaction and patient satisfaction. *Pediatrics,* 42, 855-871.

Korsch, B. M., & Negrete, V. F. (1972). Doctor-patient communication. *Scientific American,* 227(2), 66-74.

Kreps, G. L., & Thornton, B. C. (1984). *Health communication.* New York: Longman.

Leathers, D. G. (1976). *Nonverbal communication systems.* Boston: Allyn and Bacon.

Leebov, W. (1988). *Service excellence: The customer relations strategy for health care.* Chicago: American Hospital Association.

Ley, P. (1983). Patients' understanding and recall in clinical communication failure. In D. Pendelton & and J. Hasler (Eds.), *Doctor-patient communication.* (pp. 89-107). London: Academic Press.

Ley, P., & Spellman, M. S. (1967). *Communication with the patient.* London: Staples Press.

Lynch, J. J. (1977). *The broken heart: The medical consequences of loneliness.* New York: Basic Books.

Meichenbaum, D., & Turk, D. C. (1987). *Facilitating treatment adherence.* New York: Plenum.

Mehrabian, A. (1971). *Silent messages.* Belmont, CA: Wadsworth.

Northouse, P. G., & Northouse, L. L. (1985). *Health communication: A handbook for health professionals.* Englewood Cliffs, NJ: Prentice-Hall.

Okrent, D. (1987). You and the doctor: Striving for a better relationship. *The New York Times Magazine,* (March 29), 20-21, 92-94.

Omachonu, V. K. (1990). Quality of care and the patient: New criteria for evaluation. *Health Care Management Review,* 15(4), 43-50.

Pascoe, G. C. (1983). Patient satisfaction in primary health care: A literature review and analysis. *Evaluation and Program Planning,* 6, 185-210.

Pendleton, D., & Hasler, J. (1983). *Doctor-patient communication.* London: Academic Press,

President's Commission for the Study of Ethical Problems in Medicine and Biomedical and Behavoral Research (1982). *Making health care decisions: Vol. 1.* Washington, DC: U.S. Government Printing Office.

Roethlisberger, F. J., & Dickson, W. J. (1941). *Management and the worker.* Cambridge, MA: Harvard University Press.

Rosenthal, R., & Jacobson, L. (1968). *Pygmalion in the classroom.* New York: Holt, Rinehart and Winston.

Rost, K., Carter, W., & Inui, T. (1989). Introduction of information during the initial medical visit: Consequences for patient follow-through with physician recommendations for medication. *Social Science and Medicine,* 28(4), 315-321.

Ruben, B. D. (1985). *The bottomline: A patient relations training program.* Morristown, NJ: Morristown Memorial Hospital.

Ruben, B. D. (1986). *Patient perceptions of quality of care: Survey Results. No. 2.* Unpublished Report.

Ruben, B. D. (1987). *Patient perceptions of quality of care: Survey Results. No. 3.* Unpublished Report.

Ruben, B. D. (1990a). The health caregiver-patient relationship: Pathology, etiology, treatment. In E. B. Ray & L. Donohew (Ed.), *Communication and health: Systems and applications* (pp. 51-68). Hillsdale, NJ: Lawrence Erlbaum, 1989.

Ruben, B. D. (1990b). *Building effective client and colleague relationships: Lessons from patients, the literature and the pet shop.* Paper presented at the general session of the Annual Conference of the Mid-Atlantic College Health Association, Seven Springs Center, Champion, PA, October, 1990.

Ruben, B. D. (1991) *Stories patients tell: The role of interpersonal communication in patients' narratives on memorable health care encounters and experiences.* Paper presented at the Annual Conference of the International Communication Association, May, 1991, Chicago.

Ruben, B. D. (1992a). *Communication and human behavior.* 3rd ed.. Englewood Cliffs, NJ: Prentice Hall.

Ruben, B. D. (1992b) Critical health care encounters and experiences from the patient perspective: The role of interpersonal communication. *Health Communication.* In preparation.

Ruben, B. D., & Bowman, J. C. (1986). Patient satisfaction: Critical issues in the theory and design of patient relations training. *Journal of health care Education and Training,* 1(1), 1-5.

Ruben, B. D., Christensen, D., & Guttman, N. (1990). *College health service: A qualitative analysis of the patient perspective.* Unpublished Report.

Ruben, B. D., Guttman, N. & Christensen, D. (1992) *The college health service experience: What patients remember.* Paper presented at the Annual Conference of the International Communication Association, May, 1992, Miami.

Ruben, B. D. & Guttman, N. (1992). *Caregiver-patient communication: Readings.* Dubuque, IA: Kendall-Hunt.

Ruben, B. D., & Ruben, J. M. (1988). *Patient perceptions of quality of care: Survey Results. No. 5.* Unpublished Report.

Ruben, B. D., & Ruben, J. M. (1987). *Patient perceptions of quality of care: Survey Results.* No. 4. Unpublished Report.

Ruben, B. D., Zakahi, W. and Kreps, G. (1985). *Patient perceptions of quality of care: Survey Results. No. 1.* Unpublished Report.

Sacks, O. (1984). *A leg to stand on.* New York: Harper & Row.

Sanders, P. (1990). Patient relations for malpractice claim prevention. *Report of the MMIC Risk Management Committee.*

Seaver, W. B. (1973). Effects of naturally induced teacher expectancies. *Journal of Personality and Social Psychology,* 28(3), 333-342.

Shorter, E. (1985). *Bedside manners: The troubled history of doctors and patients.* New York: Simon and Schuster.

Siegel, B. S. (1986). *Love, medicine and miracles.* New York: Harper & Row.

Siegel, J. M. (1990). Stressful life events and the use of physician services among the elderly: The moderating role of pet ownership. *Journal of Personality and Social Psychology,* 58(6), 1081-1086.

Spitzberg, B. H. & Cupach, W. R. (1984). *Interpersonal communication competence.* Beverly Hills, CA: Sage.

Stewart, M., & Roter, D. (1989). *Communicating with medical patients.* Newbury Park, CA: Sage.

The quality imperative. *Business Week,* October 25, 1991.

Thompson, T. L. (1986). *Communication for health professionals.* Lanham, MD: University Press of America.

U.S. Department of Health and Human Services (1973). *Report of the Secretary's Commission on Medical Malpractice.* Washington, D.C. GPO.

Waitzkin, H. B. (1991). *The politics of medical encounters.* New Haven: Yale University Press.

Waitzkin, H. (1984). Doctor-patient communication: Clinical implications of social scientific research. *Journal of the American Medical Association,* 252(17), 2441-2446.

Waitzkin, H. (1985) Information giving in medical care. *Journal of Health and Social Behavior.* 26, 81-101.

Waitzkin, H. B. (1986). Research on doctor-patient communication: Implications for practice. *The Internist,* (August), 7-10.

Ware, J. E., Jr. & Davies, A. R. (1983). Behavioral consequences of consumer dissatisfaction with medical care. *Evaluation and Program Planning,* 6, 291-297.

Wertz, D. C., Sorenson, J. R., & Heeren, T. C. (1988). Communication in health professional-lay encounters. In B. D. Ruben (Ed.), *Information and Behavior: Volume 2* (pp. 329-342). New Brunswick, NJ: Transaction.

Wilmot, W. W. (1987). *Dyadic communication.* 3rd. ed. New York: Random House.

Woolley, F. R., Kane, R. L., & Associates (1978). The effects of doctor-patient communication on satisfaction and outcomes of care. *Social Science and Medicine,* 12, 123-128.

Appendix

CRITICAL INCIDENTS IN
PHYSICIAN-PATIENT RELATIONSHIPS

"Melanoma"

Consider the following situation, the perspectives of the people involved, the quality of clinical and communication treatment provided, and alternative approaches and strategies that might have minimized some of the difficulties:

I

When drying off from a shower, Jim – a thirteen-year old boy – noticed that the mole on his hip seemed larger than he remembered it being. He told his mother about it, and they made an appointment to visit the family doctor.

The doctor examined Jim and left the room without saying a word. He returned moments later accompanied by all the other doctors who were in that morning. They asked Jim to lay on his back, and began examining his lymph nodes. Jim did not know what they were doing, but knew something was wrong because the mole in question was on his hip. His mother broke the silence by saying, "Are you going to send us to someone else? and they responded "Yes." They all left, and one physician went into his private office to use the telephone.

In a few minutes, Jim's mother was taken to a separate room where they told her they were sending her to a plastic surgeon immediately because they felt sure it was a melanoma. She began to visibly shake and asked him what she would say to Jim, as he had already asked her on the way there if it could be skin cancer. He said it was absolutely necessary to be frank with kids Jim's age. They felt if you do not level with them from the start, you will have a lot of anger to deal with later. They were so certain that Jim's mole was a melanoma that they felt it best to have him prepared.

Jim's mom returned to Jim who was now visibly frightened. The physician told Jim he would be going to see the surgeon in a few hours. Jim said "Do you think I have cancer?" His answer was, "it appears that way to us, but you will have to see this surgeon and get it

99

removed." Jim was fighting back tears and the doctor walked out. When Jim and his mom got outside the office, Jim just began banging his fist on the brick wall and crying. His mother tried unsuccessfully to calm him.

II

An appointment was made for a visit to the plastic surgeon. When the plastic surgeon arrived, he began explaining how he had planned on leaving on vacation the next day and it was his policy not to operate on anyone the day before leaving town. As he began to examine it, the mother began to plead with him to remove it before leaving on vacation. He then turned to Jim and his mother and said,"You know, if it is what we think it is, it doesn't matter if we take it off in two days or two months, it is already too late." He was standing right beside Jim when he said that.

He then examined it further and said although it appeared to be a very advanced melanoma, he had a gut feeling Jim just might luck out and that it might be some type of vascular lesion. He explained he had nothing to base it on except a feeling he got when pressing on it very hard. Jim and his mother were told to return the next afternoon for surgery.

III

The pediatrician called after returning home to see what had happened. When Jim's mom explained that the plastic surgeon could not do it that day, but had agreed to put off his vacation to do it the next day, the pediatrician said, "You mean you are going to let them wait another 24 hours before getting that thing off?"

The surgery was performed on a Friday and the doctor knew the family was very concerned, so he called the pathologist while they were in his office and asked for a rush on the biopsy. Jim's mother agreed to carry that specimen to the pathologist herself, and was assured that they would have an answer on Monday. The plastic surgeon would be on vacation then, but said he would call at home himself, as he would not allow the results to be transmitted by anyone else. He explained that he had taken an extra area of skin surrounding the mole and gone very deep; if it was a melanoma, they needed to count surfaces for depth.

IV

All day Monday Jim and his family waited for the call. When it didn't come by 6:00 pm, they called the surgeon's phone number and got the answering service, and eventually were connected to a nurse. She said she would contact the doctor on vacation and call us back. His message back to Jim and his family (via the nurse) was that the biopsy was not complete yet. All they could think was that it must have been positive and that they were counting those surfaces. Jim's mother tried to tell him why it hadn't yet come back and not to worry – almost an impossible task.

The next day the family called the hospital lab directly out of pure frustration, and were told that the biopsy was complete but that only their doctor could be told the results. Jim's mother called the pediatrician and began begging him to call the hospital, only to discover he had already called hours earlier and knew it was benign. For him, it was like a dead issue.

Within the hour, the surgeon called from his vacation to report the biopsy results. After telling him they already knew, Jim's mother asked him what he thought had happened. He had no explanation as to what had happened and said we would probably never know.

Upon giving Jim the "good" news, it became apparent that Jim had really resigned himself to expecting a "bad" report. Although he was thrilled with the results, he was left with the many questions, and the fears and uncertainties lingered.

V

Jim and his mother went to the pediatrician several days later for Jim's allergy shot. The custom is for allergy-shot patients to get their own charts from a special file and give them to the nurse. The last entry on Jim's which he read as he walked toward the nurse – was: "Malignant melanoma. No nodes found. Future uncertain."

Although his mother knew an update should have been made, the entry made a real impact on Jim. His mother was determined that someone should give him an explanation of what had happened to him. Jim's mother spoke to two of the older members of the practice about the situation. One began questioning the biopsy, and said he thought it should have been sent to another lab in Washington. That left Jim's mother wondering if the results truly were valid. The second said to bring Jim in and he would try to explain it. He commented that he would never have handled the situation the way his colleague did. He said that was a case of "youth vs. experience."

He explained to him that what had happened was probably due to an excessive amount of hormone activity that interacted in an inappropriate way and caused the change to occur. Jim's concern was whether it would happen again. He told Jim he would probably be at risk as long as he was in puberty and the thing that caused his change was indeed the same thing that would cause a melanoma.

V I

A few months later during a visit for an allergy shot, Jim and his mother ran into the original pediatrician that had handled the case. When he saw Jim, he came toward him laughing, saying, "Gee, you really had us scared around here." Jim didn't respond.

"One More Patient"

Consider the following situation, the perspective each person brings to the encounter, communication dynamics that are likely to develop, and strategies that might help to overcome some of the problems that are likely to occur:

Patient: You have been coming to the health center for the past two weeks suffering from an acute infection. It has been one test after another and still you have not been given a diagnosis. You are angry and scared. You don't know what is wrong and you feel your condition is deteriorating.

Last night was particularly upsetting. You had been waiting all day for your physician to call, but he never did. You were unable to sleep - tossing & turning. At 5:15 a.m. you noticed your bed is soaking wet. You take your temperature and find it is 102 degrees. Feeling more and more frustrated you call the health center number to be told your primary physician will not be able to see you until late in the day. You finally accept an appointment for 4:30 p.m. You decide to arrive at 4:00 p.m., hoping to be seen earlier.

Nurse: You are a Registered Nurse working at the health center. Due to recent short-staffing you have been working overtime every day which is causing major problems with your family.

It has been another extremely busy day. The last patient appointment is a patient suspected as having AIDS who is considered by the staff to be very demanding and confrontive. You had hoped to get off work on time today, but once again the schedule has backed up. At 5:00 p.m. the receptionist tells you that the last patient has been waiting for an hour and is having a temper tantrum in the waiting room.

Physician: This has been a particularly exhausting week. Your second child, only two weeks old seems to have her days and nights mixed up. You and your wife are sleeping only an hour a night. In addition you are covering for another primary physician, a good friend, who is seriously ill.

The nurse has done nothing but complain all week about having to work overtime. You suspect that if she were more competent the overtime would have been unnecessary. After what seems like an endless stream of patients you now have to tell the final patient of the day that his diagnosis of AIDS has been confirmed.

You look at the chart and see that you have one last patient waiting to be seen.

"Tests"

Consider the following situation, the perspectives of each person, and the probable consequences of the encounter:

Patient: You arrive at 10:00 A.M., on time for out-patient tests. You have an important meeting elsewhere at noon. You inform the staff member at the desk of the appointment, and you are assured that there should be no problem.

An hour passes, and you haven't yet been called in for the test. No explanation is provided by the staff. At 11:15, you approach the desk in frustration, and explain that you will have to reschedule the test because you must leave for an appointment. As you depart, you overhear a staff member at the desk say, "Well, one less patient to see today!"

Receptionist: You're over-booked for tests today, and everything is running behind. The 10:00 a.m. patient arrives for his appointment, tells you he's concerned about the time. It seems he has some other appointment at noon. You tell him that he shouldn't worry. At around 11:00, the man comes up to the desk to tell you he's decided to leave for his other appointment. That's certainly his choice. You start to ask about rescheduling, but he seems too preoccupied with his other appointment to hear you.

Topic Index